I AM NOT SICK
I Don't Need Help!

How to Help
Someone
Accept
Treatment

20th Anniversary Edition

Xavier Amador, Ph.D.

Vida Press, New York
2020

I AM NOT SICK, I DON'T NEED HELP!
Xavier Amador

Copyright © 2000-2020 by Vida Press, L.L.C.

Also available in other translations, an audiobook from Audible.com, and as an eBook. On the web: www.VidaPress.com

Amador, Xavier, 1959 -
I AM NOT SICK, I DON'T NEED HELP!
How to Help Someone Accept Treatment.
20th Anniversary Edition / Xavier Amador.

ISBN-13: 978-0-9852067-0-3

for
Henry, Tatiana, Robinson,
and Aniceto Amador

Contents

Foreword

by Pete Earley (2nd Edition)

How would you feel, Dad, if someone you loved killed himself?

I was rushing my college age son, Mike, to an emergency room when he asked me that question. He was seeing secret messages in bumper stickers and experiencing rapid mood swings. When we reached the hospital, I felt a tremendous sense of relief. *The doctors there would know what to do!*

Four hours later, a doctor finally appeared and after briefly questioning Mike, declared there was nothing he could do to help him. Mike was convinced that he wasn't sick and he refused to take anti-psychotic medication.

Because the doctor did not believe Mike was an "imminent danger," either to himself or others, my son was turned away even though he was clearly delusional.

During the next forty-eight hours, Mike decompensated. Only another parent can really understand how agonizing it is to stand by and watch your child slip further and further into a mental abyss. I tried, of course, to intervene. I told Mike that his anti-psychotic medicine would help him think more clearly. But he told me there wasn't anything wrong with the way he was thinking. I tried to show him that he was having delusions, but he disagreed. Finally, I begged him to take his pills. "Please, please, just do it for me!" But he wouldn't. "I'm not sick," he kept repeating. After hours and hours of exhausting conversations, I demanded that he take his medication or leave the house. That threat only made the situation worse. Afraid of what might happen to him on the street, I backed down. The next morning, when Mike caught me spiking his breakfast cereal with his medicine, he became enraged.

Forty-eight hours later, Mike was in police custody. He had slipped outside one morning and broken into a house to take a bubble bath because he felt dirty. Luckily, the homeowners were out of town. It took six officers to subdue him. Mike was charged with two felony crimes.

Uncertain what to do, I contacted the National Alliance on Mental Illness (NAMI), the nation's largest grassroots mental health organization, and a volunteer there urged me to read Dr. Xavier Amador's book, *I Am Not Sick, I Don't Need Help!*

When I did, I was amazed. Just about everything that I had done to help Mike had been wrong. Rather than calming the situation, my actions had driven a wedge between Mike and me. I had not Listened to him, not Empathized with him, certainly not Agreed with him and finally had not formed a Partnership with him. Those are the four guiding principles behind LEAP, an acronym that Dr. Amador has coined to help teach parents and others how to better communicate with their mentally ill loved ones. When I was arguing with Mike, I had felt frustrated and overwhelmed. In Dr. Amador's book, I found a simple-to-understand blueprint for parents, siblings, children, and friends to follow. While I was reading Dr. Amador's book, I also realized I was not alone. Others had faced the very same situation that I had encountered with Mike.

I discovered that Dr. Amador's advice came from years of experience as a clinical psychologist. His academic and professional credentials were impressive. He had served as a professor of psychiatry at Columbia University, as Director of Research at NAMI, and Director of Psychology at the New York State Psychiatric Institute. He had worked as an NBC News consultant, appeared on countless television news shows, been quoted regularly in the media, and had been called on by the National Institute of Mental Health, Veteran's Administration, and U.S. Justice Department for advice. Dr. Amador also had served as an expert witness in high-profile cases, including the Theodore Kaczynski "Unabomber" trial, the Elizabeth Smart kidnapping, and the Zacarias Moussaoui "Twentieth Hijacker" case.

But it was another tidbit from Dr. Amador's background that really caught my eye. His brother, Enrique, has schizophrenia. This was important to me, because it meant Dr. Amador not only had professional experience, but also a personal stake in his research. One of the reasons why he had developed LEAP was to help him find ways to better understand his own brother.

Eventually, my son was sentenced to two years of probation and during that period, Mike followed the rules. He attended therapy, participated in group sessions and took his medication. But several months after Mike's court-imposed sanctions ended, signs of his illness began to resurface. I was stunned when I discovered that Mike had stopped taking his medication. Despite everything that we had gone through, he had, once again, quit taking his pills. My first impulse was to confront him. *How could you do this again? Haven't you learned anything?* But my wife reminded me of Dr. Amador's book. Using LEAP, she was able to work out an agreement that soon had him back on his medication and into treatment.

In this new edition, Dr. Amador updates his groundbreaking book. He explains how "unawareness" of a mental illness is a *symptom* brought on by the disease. It is *not* a choice that an ill person makes. He gives practical advice about how families and doctors can bridge the gap created by the federal Health Insurance Portability and Accountability Act (HIPAA) that frequently prevents loved ones from being informed and involved in treatment. He summarizes state commitment laws, using simple-to-understand terms to explain the legal complexities. Since releasing his first book, Dr. Amador has delivered more than 300 lectures and conducted hundreds of LEAP workshops. He has taken information from those sessions and added it to this edition. These include model scripts that suggest specific phrases to use and NOT to use. Being able to refer to these passages is much like having Dr. Amador in your hip pocket.

The needs of every individual who has a mental illness are unique. But regardless of that person's specific problems, the basics that Dr. Amador teaches help readers improve their communication skills, help develop trust, and help turn combative situations into cooperative ones.

One night while Dr. Amador was autographing books, a man approached him empty handed. He had left his dog-eared copy at home, he explained, but had stood in line anyway because he wanted to shake the hand of the doctor who had, as he put it, "given me my son back."

I feel the same way.

‖‖

Pete Earley is the author of *Crazy: A Father's Search through America's Mental Health Madness*. He is a former investigative journalist for the *Washington Post* and the author of several *New York Times* best-selling books.

Preface to the 20th Anniversary Edition
Xavier Amador (2020)

This little book, which started out as a labor of love, continues to grow in its reach to family members, doctors, nurses, therapists, criminal justice professionals and policy-makers. It has been translated into French, Spanish, Hungarian, Chinese, Arabic, Czechoslovakian, Polish, Japanese, Swedish and other languages around the world. I did not revise this book because of its success—I revised it because of what was missing in the earlier editions. Countless readers have asked me to give them more guidance on how to use LEAP in their specific situations and especially, on how to get to partnering.

To address this request for guidance, together with two co-founders (one being my daughter Tatiana), I founded the LEAP Foundation for Research to Practice: see www.LFRP.org. This nonprofit public charity has trained thousands in the use of LEAP and has gone further by training trainers so that hundreds of LEAP trainers can now be found across the U.S.A. Still, this book was not addressing the need, the complaint, for more advice on how to use the LEAP approach. So, in addition to much updated research which has been included in the pages that follow, a more robust and wise guide to learning and using LEAP appears in this book.

There is one more reason a revision was needed. In addition to beefing up the LEAP chapters so readers could more quickly get to partnering, the book needed to reflect the way LEAP has been used by families and in the field. More and more professionals and family members have been using both this book and the LEAP approach to deal with persons caught in the throes of addiction. This trend over the years had not surprised me. I have been hearing stories of how LEAP helped in the case of addictions for twenty years now. Also, LEAP is based in part on a well-studied approach to addiction called Motivational Interviewing. You will find in the pages ahead, more direct emphasis on addiction, unawareness of addiction and how to use LEAP to help someone with addiction accept treatment.

It was now almost forty years ago (in 1981) that I first learned how my natural instinct to confront denial of illness head-on led to disaster. My brother had just come home after his first hospitalization for schizophrenia. The medicine he had been given brought him back to the reality I knew, but within a day of his getting home, I found the pills in the garbage can. Naturally, I asked him why he'd thrown them out.

"I'm okay now. I don't need it anymore," he explained. Since this ran counter to everything he was told in the hospital, I made a point of reminding him.

"But the doctor said you're probably going to have to take this medicine for the rest of your life. You can't stop taking it!"

"He didn't say that."

"Sure, he did! I was at the family meeting, remember?"

"No. He said I had to take it while I was in the hospital."

"Then why did he give you a supply of medicine to take home?" I argued, trying to prove him wrong.

"That was just in case I got sick again. I'm fine now."

"No. That's not what he said."

"Yes, it is."

"Why are you being so stubborn? You know I'm right!" I said.

"It's my business. Leave me alone."

"When you got sick, it became everyone's business. And besides, I'm worried."

"You don't have to worry about me. I'm fine."

"You're fine now, but you won't be if you don't stay on the medicine."

"That's not what the doctor said!"

"Then let's call him and I'll prove it!"

"I don't want to talk about it! Just leave me alone," he said as he walked away.

With every dose of "reality" I tried to give him, Henry countered with more denials. And with every go-round we both became angrier and angrier.

I thought he was being stubborn and immature. My accusations and threats to prove him wrong made him angry and defensive. My natural instinct to confront his denial was completely ineffective and made things worse. We got caught in a cycle of more confrontation and denials (what I call the denial dance), which pushed us farther apart. The end result was always that he walked away angry. And then he would relapse and end up back in the hospital.

The solution I came upon, with my brother and then with the patients I worked with, is one I have shared with you in this new book. I have given over one thousand talks and workshops on the problem of denial and the 7 LEAP tools offered in this book. LEAP seminars have been presented all over the United States, in many cities in France, Belgium, Australia, New Zealand, Hungary, Croatia, the United Kingdom, Portugal, Turkey, the Gulf Community of Countries (GCC), and Spain.

And now with the launch of the nonprofit LEAP Foundation, my hope is to bring LEAP to families, mental health practitioners, and criminal justice professionals throughout the U.S.A. (see: www.LFRP.org).

I end here, again, with a quote from my foreword to the first edition, published in 2000: "After my lecture [about the research on poor insight] I was surrounded at the podium for nearly two hours, speaking with family members who wanted advice and a greater understanding of why their loved ones refused to accept help. The yearning of these people to learn more and to talk to someone who understood their frustration was enlightening. I was also struck by the realization that the scientific advances with which I was so familiar hadn't yet reached many of the people who would benefit most from what has been learned. That is why I wrote this book."

I AM NOT SICK
I Don't Need Help!

Introduction

If you are reading *I Am Not Sick, I Don't Need Help!* it is probably because you have a serious problem. You are trying to reach someone with serious mental illness or addiction who is in "denial" and, most likely, is refusing treatment and relapsing. Or, if he is in treatment, he is dropping out again and again. You've tried various strategies that haven't worked and you're seeking information about how you can help him or her to get help. You may be a loved one of such a person, or a mental health practitioner, or a criminal justice professional (police, corrections, probation, judge, etc.). Whomever you are in your approach to this problem, this book was written for you.

In this book I write both about persons with serious mental illness and those with addiction. These problems are not mutually exclusive. Although most of this book focuses on examples of persons with mental illness rather than addiction, the solutions offered can work for either. Indeed, the LEAP approach is used regularly with patients in recovery from addiction. Nevertheless, to be faithful to the lineage of this book, the examples are nearly all focused on persons with mental illness. I invite the reader primarily interested in helping someone with addiction to not be deterred as the communication techniques I give here apply to persons struggling with addiction and in denial of their substance abuse problems (alcohol or drugs).

The first part of this book provides information about the nature and scope of the problem you are about to tackle. Some of you may be tempted to skip this section and go directly to the chapters on LEAP (Part II of this book)—a communication strategy designed to win the trust of persons who lack insight for the purpose of becoming a "friend" whose advice they will follow (e.g., to accept treatment, supportive housing, rehab, and other services). I have no problem with that and encourage you to do so if your situation is urgent. Or, if the situation is even *more* urgent, you may want to turn directly to Part III, where I provide practical guidance about when and how to secure "assisted treatment" (inpatient or outpatient involuntary treatment). In my mind, skipping ahead would be an appropriate use of this book. If you do that, however, I strongly urge you—after things have settled down—to go back and read the three chapters that make up Part I.

The information in Part I is vital for several reasons. First, it will help you to understand what the newest research has shown about the causes of what may seem to you nothing more than pure stubbornness on the part of the person you are trying to help. Too often, people with these disorders feel that we are their enemies. (I am speaking both as a therapist and as a family member.) From their perspective, we are adversaries and detractors—definitely not allies. Meanwhile, we scratch our heads and wonder why they seem unable or unwilling to accept the help we offer. In this context, it is not surprising that the relationship often becomes adversarial. However, once you understand that the mentally ill and addicted person's refusal to accept treatment typically results from a brain dysfunction that is beyond his control, you will see why you shouldn't take it personally or blame him for what appears to be deliberate denial.

Countless times following lectures I have given to professional and lay audiences (family members and consumers/patients), someone will come up and tell me that knowledge of the new research has helped to alleviate guilt. Just as often, I am told that this information helps to diminish blame and anger directed toward the mentally ill person who is refusing help. If you are feeling angry and blaming the person you are trying to help (both common and natural feelings), you will be much less effective in what you are trying to accomplish, and your task will be an unhappy adversarial endeavor rather than a positive collaboration.

Just as importantly, however, you will learn why it's so important for you to keep trying. The research indicates that the sooner someone receives treatment, the better his prognosis, the less frequently he will be hospitalized, and the shorter his hospital stays will be. It's often difficult to maintain your resolve when you are dealing with someone who wants no part of what you are offering, so knowing just how vital treatment is will help you to persevere.

Once you know the nature of the problem and why you so urgently need to address it, you will be better prepared to understand and implement the new approach to dealing with poor insight and treatment refusal described in the second part of the book. The techniques you will learn—LEAP—are not only informed by the research on insight and treatment adherence (i.e., participation in treatment) you will already have read about, but are also based on the results of recent *placebo controlled studies* and on my own clinical experience working with patients and families and supervising other therapists.

I can't guarantee that LEAP will definitely eliminate treatment refusal in the person you're trying to help, but I can promise that if you faithfully follow the guidelines I give, they will help lower tension, increase trust, and greatly increase the likelihood that the person you are trying to help will follow your advice. And if my previous experience and the published research are any indication, chances are good that you can make a very positive difference.

During the time you are working on the problem, you may face the difficult dilemma of countless other family members and therapists: whether or not to force treatment by using the involuntary commitment laws in your state. Doing this can sometimes be a vital part of the treatment process, but it is most effective when it is done in a way that ultimately strengthens your alliance with the person you're helping rather than destroying it. The third part of this book focuses on the question of when to "commit or not commit" someone to hospital or outpatient treatment against his or her will. You will learn not only the nuts and bolts of how to seek commitment to the hospital, but also how to cope with the difficult feelings this kind of intervention raises for everyone involved. My main goal is to show you how to deal with the accusations of betrayal you will likely encounter, the guilt you may feel and, most importantly, how to use the commitment itself to build trust and a sense of teamwork with the very person you forced into treatment.

Too often, inpatient treatment is crisis-driven and, hence, short-sighted. You can, however, build upon the trust and gains you have achieved after the person is discharged from the hospital, and I'll be providing you with strategies for doing just that.

Finally, Part IV of the book ties it all together. You learn, in a brief chapter, the theoretical and scientific basis of LEAP, about other forms of psychotherapy that have been found to be effective in lowering symptoms and how the research argues strongly for a revision of how we make diagnoses in patients with extreme denial. In short, I argue that we must assess and document whether the person has awareness of his or her illness so we can design a treatment plan that makes sense.

In the last chapter, I tell you about Henry's death. More accurately, I tell you about his life and his relationships with his girlfriend, friends, caseworker and his younger brother — me.

My intention is for you to draw inspiration and motivation from this chapter as LEAP saved our relationship and gave us many years of joy and hope. In this chapter, I hope to share with you something about Henry's remarkable selflessness.

The final section is a concise summary of all the major interventions described in the book. It is quite literally a LEAP "cheat sheet" in that it will help you to easily remember the essential tools to convince someone in "denial" to accept treatment and services and, more importantly, to accept your friendship and support.

Finally, I encourage all family members to investigate and become involved with one of the family-advocacy groups and consumer organizations I list in the Resources section (e.g., NAMI, AL-ANON). There are many reasons to do so, not the least of which is to feel less alone and more supported in your quest to better the life of your mentally ill relative. These organizations will also help you to feel less ashamed and embarrassed about having a mentally ill person in your family. These feelings are unwarranted and will only hinder you in your attempts to help your loved one.

For too many years, I was ashamed about my brother, who had schizophrenia. Despite knowing that he suffered from a brain disorder and that I had nothing to feel ashamed about, I avoided such organizations and kept his illness a secret from my colleagues. It was only after talking with people like myself that I was able to stop feeling ashamed. Because of my own experience, I would certainly understand if you don't feel that you are ready to attend any kind of meeting or conference about mental illness. It is ironic and sad that the instinct not to talk about family problems keeps many of us from receiving the support and information we need to solve those problems.

However, you can benefit from such organizations even if you still feel hesitant about getting involved. You don't have to attend a single meeting to learn from their websites or request other literature offered by these groups. I have learned much from these organizations and have found great comfort in knowing not only that there are many other families like mine but also that there are forces at work to change mental health laws, fund research, and improve treatments.

For therapists who read this book, I aim to give you hope that you can reach your patients/clients with serious mental illness and/or addiction who don't think they're ill and refuse your help. Whether you are a mental health professional or a family member, this book will help to dispel the despair that sometimes makes you want to turn your head and look the other way. It will give you renewed hope that you can make a big difference.

Part I

The Truth about Denial of Illness

Knowledge is happiness, because to have knowledge — broad, deep knowledge — is to know true ends from false, and lofty things from low.

—Helen Keller—

Whilst part of what we perceive comes through our senses from the object before us, another part (and it may be the larger part) always comes from our own mind.

The fact that the brain is the one immediate bodily condition of the mental operations is indeed so universally admitted nowadays that I need spend no more time in illustrating it, but will simply postulate it and pass on.

—William James—
The Principles of Psychology,
Volume I, 1890, Foreword

1

We Are Not Alone

"I am not sick! I don't need help!"
Henry Amador, as shouted at the author

"He has horrible delusions about us and won't talk to the family. He would rather be homeless than accept our help. He's living on the street — we don't know where."
Pete and Linda, as told to the author

"My brother is so ill. He's refused to take the medication. We've tried to talk him into it," said April Callahan, sister of Russell Weston, who is charged with having shot two guards at the U.S. Capitol. *"He just wouldn't do it,"* added his mother, Arbah Weston. *"What are we going to do with a 41-year-old man? You can't throw him in the car."*
AP wire, July 26, 1998

"There was [this] sick person [who] broke into David Letterman's house. That was her illness. She had an aversion to treatment and to admitting that she had a problem."
Anna-Lisa Johanson, as told to the author

"My mother wanted us to camp out on his land and convince him to get help. As far as he was concerned we had the problem, not him."
David Kaczynski, brother of the confessed "Unabomber"
Ted Kaczynski, as told to the author

"After Jeff's last manic episode, I thought he'd finally realized he needed to stay on the medicine. But last week, he stopped taking his lithium again. He says he's better now and doesn't need it anymore!"
Julia, as told to the author

9

We are not alone. I use "we" instead of "you" because I have met countless families just like my own—and yours—estranged from a loved one who has no clue they have mental illness or addiction. And what of the families who don't consider themselves as part of the "we" I just described? Whether they realize it or not, they see their family's story in the headlines: Millions of people with mental illness and addictions are in denial that they are ill and, therefore, refuse treatment. Those of us who are related to such persons can't help but see ourselves and our loved ones reflected in those headlines. Pete, Linda and Julia's predicament, which was never the focus of any news story, highlights a problem encountered by about 11 million U.S. families and tens of millions more from around the world whose names never appear in the press. It is, in fact, a far more common scenario than those involving violence or suicide, which are, of course, the ones we read about. But just like the more infamous examples cited above, Pete and Linda's and Julia's loved ones do not think they are ill and don't accept treatment. Their denial and refusal may not lead to infamy, but they will almost certainly lead to worsening illness, a life derailed and endangered, lost opportunities, and ruined relationships with loved ones.

Some people with bipolar disorder, schizophrenia and addictions think of their illness as something that is part of their past. It came and it went. For a short time, Jeff acknowledged he had an illness and took the medication prescribed for it. But after things got better, he decided he didn't need to keep taking the lithium. For Jeff, lithium was medicine to treat his mental illness in the same way that antibiotics are medicines for an infection. When the bottle is empty, you are cured. In reality, the better comparison is that lithium is for bipolar disorder what insulin is for diabetes, medicine that needs to be taken every day to prevent a relapse or even death. Because both bipolar disorder and schizophrenia are almost as lethal as addictions (10% to 15%

who suffer from these disorders die from suicide), this analogy is particularly apt. Even though Jeff took his medication only sporadically, he was still a step ahead of the game, because many people with serious mental illness[1] never acknowledge that they're ill and refuse all forms of treatment.

David Kaczynski, the brother of Theodore Kaczynski, the "Unabomber," told me that even though his brother had terrorized the nation for two decades, the Kaczynski family had received countless letters expressing support, understanding, and condolences from people who were related to someone with a serious mental illness. Like David and his mother, they had experienced the helplessness and heartache associated with caring about someone who was in denial about having a mental illness. In fact, I was one of those letter writers. Like the others, I saw my own situation reflected in that of the Kaczynski family. I've just been luckier because my brother Henry, like the overwhelming majority of people with these illnesses, was never violent.

Far more common than the tragedies that make the headlines are those that test the bonds of family and the moral resolve of the therapists and criminal justice professionals who are entrusted with the care of our loved ones. When once again a bottle of medication is found in the trash or stuffed under a mattress, when we are told to mind our own business or that we are the crazy ones, when yet another doctor's appointment is missed, we all come one step closer to throwing our hands up in despair. Sometimes, whether or not we walk away, our *loved ones*[2] do. They disappear

---

1 Many mental disorders can be very serious (e.g., addiction, depression, anxiety, personality disorders and others). However, for the sake of brevity, I will use the term "serious mental illnesses" to refer primarily to psychotic illnesses including schizophrenia, schizoaffective disorder, bipolar disorder (formerly "manic depression"), and addiction.

2 Since this book is written for both lay and professional readers who are trying to help someone with a serious mental illness, there are many terms I could use to refer to the person being helped (e.g., patient, consumer, family member, loved one, subject, suspect, etc.). To avoid cumbersome language, I will mostly use the terms "loved one," "family member," or "relative," from this point forward. Readers who are mental health care providers and criminal justice professionals should substitute "patient," "client," "consumer," "individual," or "suspect" (whatever is typical for your circumstance) for the familial reference.

for hours, days, weeks, and even years. My brother Henry was in the habit of disappearing for days and even hitch-hiking cross-country. Some make the headlines anonymously when they join the ranks of the homeless or incarcerated. That used to be my biggest fear.

There are approximately eleven million people in the United States with *serious mental illnesses,* and literally hundreds of millions more worldwide. The results of recent studies indicate unequivocally that about 50% of all people with these disorders don't believe they're ill and refuse services and to take the medications that have been prescribed for them. That amounts to more than five million *seriously mentally ill* Americans who don't realize they're ill. You probably already had some idea of how widespread these illnesses are, but did you ever stop and think about how many family members there are? If we count only the parents of these individuals, there are twice that number of family members! Add just one sibling or offspring, and the number becomes truly staggering. Now here's the real headline: *More than fifteen million Americans have a close relative with mental illness who is in denial and refusing treatment.*

Most studies find that about one-half of the people with serious mental illness don't take their medication. The most common reason is poor insight into illness.

In the past twenty years, there has been an explosion of research on the problem of poor insight. Among the earlier studies during this period was one conducted by my colleagues and me. We studied more than 400 patients with psychotic disorders from all over the United States. This "field trial" was conducted as part of our participation in the revision of the *Diagnostic and Statistical Manual of Mental Disorders* (DSM) conducted by the American Psychiatric Association. We measured a wide range of symptoms, including insight into various aspects of the illness and treatment. What we hoped to learn was how frequently people with a mental disorder did not realize they were ill. Our results showed that nearly 60% of the patients with schizophrenia, about 25% of those with schizoaffective disorder, and nearly 50% of subjects with bipolar disorder were unaware of being ill. This main finding has been replicated more than one hundred times in the research literature and is so widely accepted in the field nowadays that, as of the year 2000, the standard diagnostic manual used by all mental health professionals in the U.S., at that time, states that, "A majority of individuals with schizophrenia have poor insight into the fact that they have a psychotic illness..." Page, 304 (*Diagnostic and Statistical Manual of Mental Disorders, IV-TR*, American Psychiatric Association Press, 2000). As I describe in Chapter 3, the current DSM (DSM 5) goes much further in describing the negative impact this problem has on the lives of patients and the community.

When the patients enrolled in our DSM study were asked whether they had any mental, psychiatric, or emotional problems, about half answered "no." Usually the "no" was emphatic and followed by sometimes bizarre explanations as to why they were inpatients on a psychiatric ward. Explanations ranged from "because my parents brought me here" to stranger beliefs such as "I'm just here for a general physical." Whereas the majority of patients with depression and anxiety disorders actively seek treatment because they feel bad and want help, these individuals, by contrast, were unaware of having a serious mental illness. Unlike people with depression and anxiety, they never complained about "symptoms" because they didn't have any. Indeed, their main complaint was usually feeling victimized by their family, friends, and doctors who were pressuring them to accept treatment for an illness they didn't have!

We were surprised to learn that the problems with illness awareness did not stop at denial of a diagnosis. The unawareness we were documenting was severe and pervasive.

In addition, a significant percentage of those we studied were also unaware of the various signs of the illness they "suffered" from despite the fact that everyone around them could readily recognize the symptoms (e.g., thought disorder, mania, hallucinations, etc.). The pattern of pervasive unawareness of symptoms shown in the figure below was also found in all the other psychotic-disordered patients we studied (except those with psychotic depression). This was the first time anyone had looked at this issue and so we were surprised to learn that the problems with *illness awareness* did not stop at denial of a diagnosis. The unawareness we were documenting was severe and pervasive (i.e., patients were unaware of their diagnosis and unable to see even the most obvious signs and symptoms of their illness).

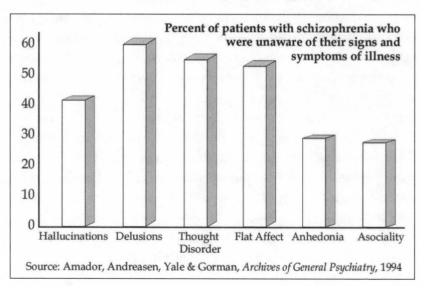

Percent of patients with schizophrenia who were unaware of their signs and symptoms of illness

Source: Amador, Andreasen, Yale & Gorman, *Archives of General Psychiatry*, 1994

To illustrate just how extreme the unawareness can be, let's look at Matt, who is a former patient of mine. As you read Matt's story, however, I want you to keep in mind that, in the chapters that follow, you'll also be learning how I was able to help him accept treatment, even though he did not believe he had a mental illness! Not surprisingly, as he was able to do that, the endless stream of conflicts with his family over his refusal to stay in treatment also came to an end.

Matt

At the time I met him, Matt was 26 years old, single, and living with his parents. He had been diagnosed with schizoaffective disorder six years before, when he first began to experience grandiose and paranoid delusions (thinking he was a special messenger from God who knew the President of the U.S.A. personally and worrying that the CIA was trying to kill him). He had disorganized speech and bizarre behaviors (wearing broken earphones that had been wrapped in aluminum foil) and was hearing voices. Although Matt was remarkably unconcerned about his obvious signs of mental illness, they gravely troubled his family, friends, and even his neighbors—who had to endure his loud speeches. He had been hospitalized on four occasions since he first became ill.

At the time of the interview you are about to read, Matt had voluntarily signed himself into the Schizophrenia Research Ward at Columbia University in New York City, where I was the Science Director. He came to us from a city hospital where he had been taken involuntarily and admitted to the psychiatric ward because his mother had called 911. Although the exact length of time is uncertain, Matt had stopped taking his medications at least six weeks before the 911 call. That night, the paranoia that had been brewing for days boiled over. Matt began to scream at his mother, accusing her of interfering with his mission from God, which, he believed, was to be His special messenger to the President. For several days, he had been frantically writing letters to the President and trying to place phone calls to the White House. Most frightening to his mother, however, was that he was hearing God's voice telling him to lock her in the closet!

By the time he arrived at Columbia, Matt had been receiving medication for one month. When I interviewed him, nearly all of his symptoms, except the delusions, had shown significant improvement. Although he still believed he was God's messenger and that the CIA was trying to kill him, he felt less urgency about these ideas and was less worried about his safety. In fact, despite his obviously poor insight into the illness, he was about to be discharged to his parents' home with a referral to an outpatient treatment program. I started the interview by asking Matt to tell me how he had come to be in the hospital.

"I think it was...I don't know the exact terms. It wasn't identified to me as of yet. I think they brought me here for a general physical. They wanted to know was I drinking, had I been smoking. I told the police that there wasn't any drinking, no smoking. It was just a mild argument we had and I believe that my mother had more seniority over what was going on. So they took me to the clinic to have the doctor determine how well off I am."

Although Matt's speech was somewhat disorganized and a touch idiosyncratic, I caught the gist of what he was trying to tell me and asked, "So when you were having an argument with your mother, someone called the police?" He nodded. "Was it your mother?"

"I think so."

"Why did your mother call the police?"

"I don't know. She wanted me to go to the hospital."

"Why did your mother want you to come to the hospital?"

"She said she didn't really want me to go to the hospital in the event that an argument like that took place, because we were discussing my use of the telephone."

"I am a little confused by what you just said," I admitted. "Why did she want you to go to a hospital?"

"We were arguing and I think she thought I was sick and needed to be checked out."

"Were you sick?"

"No. We were just arguing."

"So the police took you to the hospital."

"That's right."

"Why did the people at the hospital admit you?"

"They didn't say. A real friendly guy was there. He said, 'Don't worry, you're going to be here for a while and I'd like you to get your thoughts together,' and I've been in the hospital ever since."

"Yes. But that was in the emergency room. What kind of a ward did you go to?"

"I went to a psychiatric ward upstairs. They removed me of my clothes, and they told me I was going to stay there for a while."

"But why a psychiatric ward?"

"I think that's all they have available now because of the heavy drug and alcohol use. They may not be receiving aid for a general check-up clinic."

"Matt, now I *am* confused. Are you saying the doctors at the city hospital admitted you to a psychiatric ward for a general physical?"

"That's right," he answered, as if there were nothing unusual or upsetting about his perception of his circumstance.

"Do you see yourself as someone who didn't need to be in a psychiatric ward?" I paused. "Do you see yourself as someone without psychiatric or emotional problems of any sort?"

"That's right. But they put me through the emotional tests because of the two-party system.[3] They asked me to cooperate. So, I've been pretty much cooperating. Some of it is against my will but I can cooperate."

"You didn't want to stay. Is that right?"

"Right."

"Why did you stay?"

"I had to because of the judge. He committed me for a month."

"But after the month was up you decided to come here, to the Schizophrenia Research Ward, yes?"

"Right."

"But you feel there is nothing wrong with you?"

"That's right. My mother wanted me to come, but there's nothing wrong with me."

To say that Matt had poor insight into his illness is an understatement. Nor does it do justice to the strangeness of the beliefs he had about what was happening to him. Matt believed that police officers had restrained him and taken him to the hospital at the request of his mother simply because she had more "seniority" than he. He also believed that an emergency room physician had admitted him to a psychiatric ward for one month to get a "general physical." And what can we make of the blasé attitude he had while describing these terrible injustices? Handcuffed by the police, taken to a hospital and incarcerated against his will for a month, and he didn't threaten lawsuits or scream bloody murder? Many patients with these illnesses do exactly that, while others have the remarkable lack of distress that Matt showed.

I should make clear the fact that Matt had an average IQ. This was not an issue of low intelligence. So then, what was going on

---

3 I believe Matt is referring to the involuntary treatment law in New York at the time which required two physicians to certify (2 PC) that the person is a danger to himself or others as a result of a mental illness and requires hospitalization and evaluation.

here? Was it that Matt was embarrassed by his mental illness and didn't want to reveal the truth to me? That's possible, but if such were the case, wouldn't a less bizarre explanation have been more convincing? More importantly, however, Matt knew that I was well aware of all the details related to his hospitalization. I was, after all, the doctor assigned to his care!

As you may already have guessed, Matt was also unaware that the voices he heard were unusual. He accepted them as if they were nothing out of the ordinary and certainly nothing to be concerned about.

Imagine if *you* suddenly started hearing voices when no one was in the room. What would you do? Very likely you would be worried, and if the hallucinations recurred, you would rush to a doctor. That's what most people would do. I know—I have worked in neurological clinics with such people. (Sometimes hallucinations are among the first symptoms of a brain tumor.) But why do some people worry when they hallucinate and others don't? Is it simply denial? Is it that some people are more able to accept that they have problems while others are too frightened, proud or stubborn? Or is there some other explanation?

At this level, poor insight is clearly another symptom of the disorder, and has nothing to do with being defensive or stubborn.

In fact, Matt was *not* in denial. Instead, our research and that of other clinical scientists tells us that Matt had at least one more symptom that had not been helped by the medicine he was given. His bizarre explanations for why he was in a psychiatric hospital (for a general physical and because all the other wards were filled with drug-addicted patients) and his failure to realize that he was ill and could benefit from medicine, were not stemming from denial or pridefulness. Nor did they have anything to do with being defensive or stubborn. Rather, his poor insight into having an illness and into the benefits of treatment was clearly *another symptom of the disorder itself.* Indeed, the research you will read about in Chapter 3 explains that this type of poor insight is more readily understood as one of the *neurocognitive deficits,* or symptoms of a *brain dysfunction,* that are commonly caused by these disorders. This is very important information because only when you understand the causes of poor insight can you be effective at dealing with the refusal of treatment that it creates.

2

Staying in the Game

"Far better is it to dare mighty things, to win glorious triumphs, even though checkered by failure, than to take up ranks with those poor spirits who neither enjoy much nor suffer much, for they live in that grey twilight that knows neither victory nor defeat."

—Theodore Roosevelt—

I wouldn't blame you if you were sometimes tempted to let the problem slide. Whether you are family, friend, therapist, or police officer simply trying to help, eventually you get tired of being told, "There's nothing wrong with me—I don't need help." Often, we feel helpless.

Certainly, when the person is not causing problems and things are going generally well, it's easy to ignore the problems of denial and treatment refusal. During those times, we're tempted to sit back and wait for the next crisis to force the issue or to hope (our own form of denial) that the disease has gone away. It's always much easier to pretend the situation is not as bad as it appears because facing the reality of the illness can feel intimidating and hopeless.

Even if we know a loved one has stopped taking her medication or is continuing to use drugs and/or alcohol, if things are calm, we can't help wanting to back off a little. This is especially true when faced with personal accusations. For example, Vicky, a manic-depressive 45-year-old mother of two, told her worried husband, "I'm not sick anymore. I am not the one with the problem; you're the one with the problem! Get off my back and stop trying to control me!" And if we suspect (but don't know for sure) that a loved one has been throwing out medications or sneaking drinks, we often back off because we don't want a negative confrontation to weaken whatever trust we've managed to build up. Later, I will explain that you don't have to back off, and what you can do to build the kind of trust that will allow you to persuade a loved one to stay in treatment. But, first, I need to address the myth that in cases of serious mental illness and addiction, it is sometimes better to "let sleeping dogs lie."

As Russell Weston's mother remarked in an interview after her son shot and killed two U.S. Capitol police officers, "What are we going to do with a 41-year-old man? You can't throw him in the car and drive him to the doctor." I wouldn't be surprised if after the fact she and her husband wished they had at least tried to do exactly that, or that they'd committed their son to a hospital without his consent.

But these things are much easier said than done. In Part III, you will learn about forced treatment (a.k.a. "assisted treatment"). Still, the decision to commit someone is very personal, much like your choice to read this book and learn how to deal with denial and refusal to accept treatment. To attack the problem, you must have hope that your efforts will make a difference. Without that element of hope, it's much easier just to let events unfold as they may. Who hasn't thought that, sooner or later, another hospitalization would end the current crisis? And, when there is *no* crisis, the temptation to "let sleeping dogs lie" is even greater.

Why We Can't Let Sleeping Dogs Lie

It has always been obvious that consistent supervision and treatment help to prevent suicide, violence, homelessness, and reckless behaviors. What had not been clear until recently, however, is the very positive effect that early and consistent treatment has on the course of the illness and the hope of recovery in persons with schizophrenia and bipolar. Understanding this research will help you to make an informed decision about what to do. If you decide to tackle the problem of denial and make facilitating consistent involvement in treatment your goal, the following information will help you to keep your resolve.

Research shows that getting seriously mentally ill persons into treatment early, and keeping them there, is very important.

According to the new research, whenever someone with serious mental illness has another episode, the long-term prognosis worsens. Some scientists have gone so far as to argue that psychotic episodes[1] are toxic to the brain.

The idea is that brain cells are altered or die during and immediately following an episode of psychosis. As yet, there is no definitive evidence to corroborate this idea but there is a good deal of indirect support coming from long-term studies of the seriously mentally ill.

In one landmark study conducted at the Hillside Hospital in Queens, New York, researchers found that those individuals with schizophrenia who received treatment early and consistently had much better outcomes. The results of the study indicate that when antipsychotic drugs are given shortly after the illness first emerges and subsequent psychotic episodes are treated

---

1 Many people refer to psychotic episodes as "nervous breakdowns," but the term nervous breakdown is also sometimes used to indicate conditions other than psychosis. An episode of psychosis specifically involves hallucinations, delusions, and/or extremely disorganized thoughts and behavior.

quickly to shorten their duration, future response to treatment and prognosis is greatly improved.

Similar results were found in a follow-up study involving 276 young, seriously mentally ill persons. The researchers studied these patients during an episode of psychosis and then stayed in contact with them for up to seven-and-one-half years. The subjects who had more psychotic episodes during the early stages of the study did much worse years later. Once again, the results strongly suggest that, by limiting the number of full-blown episodes of psychosis and intervening early when the illness does flare up, patients remain higher functioning and less ill later in life.

Finally, in a 15-year follow-up study of 82 patients with schizophrenia, researchers found that delays in mental-health treatment and longer periods of psychosis led to a worse prognosis over the long run. This study is especially informative because patients were entered into the research during their very first episodes of illness.

The studies just described are but a few examples of the growing body of evidence supporting the efficacy of early intervention for patients with schizophrenia who refuse to take medication. Furthermore, research indicates that the same holds true for other serious mental illnesses including clinical depression with or without psychosis.

In the book *When Someone You Love is Depressed: How to help your loved one without losing yourself,* my co-author Dr. Laura Rosen and I review the research on treatment of depression. Most studies find that people with untreated episodes of clinical depression (i.e., those who "ride the depression out") have a much worse course of illness and more frequent bouts of depression later in life.

Other studies show that people with bipolar disorder also do worse when episodes of illness are not treated quickly and effectively. A more thorough description of this important research can be found in the first chapter of *Out of the Shadows: Confronting America's Mental Illness Crisis* by Dr. E. Fuller Torrey. Among the reasons Dr. Torrey cites for getting the seriously mentally ill medical attention are the following statistics:

- About 3 million Americans have untreated severe mental illness
- 150,000 of them are homeless
- 159,000 are incarcerated for crimes committed while unmedicated

Dr. Torrey argues that homelessness, incarceration, episodes of violence, and premature death are not necessary because we know what to do but fail to do it for economic, legal and ideological reasons. In particular, he cites our hesitation as a society to infringe on the individual rights and freedoms of our fellow citizens as a major obstacle to providing the seriously mentally ill with the medical treatment they need.

The issue he takes on is largely beyond the scope of this book, but the case he makes for getting people with serious mental illness into treatment and for finding ways to help them become active participants in their own care is directly relevant. I encourage you to read his book, especially if, by the end of this chapter, you still have doubts about the tremendously positive impact you will have when you help someone with serious mental illness accept treatment.

We must address the twin problems of poor insight and treatment refusal if we want our loved ones to have the best possible chance of recovery.

What the three studies described above make clear is that when we ignore the problem, it not only doesn't go away—it gets *worse*. We must address the twin problems of poor insight and treatment refusal if we want our loved ones to have the best possible chance of recovery. In many ways, treatment refusal can be seen as a symptom of the underlying problem of poor insight. The good news is that scientists have learned a lot in recent years about the nature and causes of poor insight in serious mental disorders, and the findings themselves suggest specific methods for dealing with the problem. Unlike some advances in research, this is information you can put to use right now.

Myths and Facts about Insight

The best place to begin is to dispel some of the myths that have been revealed by recent research. One of the most common is that in the case of mental illness having poor insight is usually a good thing. Many times at clinical conferences, a well-meaning mental health professional will say, "No wonder he's in denial. If he had insight, he might kill himself!" I, too, used to think this way. However, the new research shows that insight is usually a very good thing but, like most good things, only in moderation. In other words, insight into some aspects of the illness is usually beneficial, while other types of insight can sometimes be detrimental.

|||||||||||||||||||||||||||||||||||||||||||||||||||||||||||||||||||||||||||||||||||||||||||||||||||||||||||||||||||||||||||||||||||||||||||||||||||||||||||||

Research shows that awareness of the positive effects of medication can be more important to medication adherence than insight into the illness itself.

|||||||||||||||||||||||||||||||||||||||||||||||||||||||||||||||||||||||||||||||||||||||||||||||||||||||||||||||||||||||||||||||||||||||||||||||||||||||||||||

In 1991, my colleagues at Columbia University and I published a paper in the National Institute of Mental Health's journal *Schizophrenia Bulletin* in which we proposed several guidelines for researchers interested in studying insight. The first guideline was that insight should be measured in all its complexity. When I use the term "insight," I am referring to much more than whether or not a mentally ill person can say, "Yes, I am ill." There are various things into which one can have insight, and some types of awareness are more vital to recovery than others. For example, a person can have insight into the fact that antipsychotic medication helps him to function in society without necessarily agreeing that he's mentally ill. Research shows that awareness of the positive effects of medication can be more important to medication adherence than insight into the illness itself. I have seen patients who are aware of some of their symptoms while unaware that the voices they alone hear are a sign of illness. Others will say they're ill but don't believe they gain any benefit from taking medication despite objective evidence to the contrary. The guidelines we proposed more than twenty years ago are now widely accepted by the scientific community, and the pace of research into the problem of poor insight has increased dramatically.

The same holds true in the case of alcohol and drug abuse. One does not have to have complete insight to decide to get help. Sometimes it is enough that the person becomes aware that his or her substance abuse has caused others serious harm and that they've lost control over how much they drink/use. Insight into having the illness (e.g., I am an alcoholic) is less important than recognizing that life is spiraling out of the person's control because of their substance use.

Whether we are talking about psychiatric illness or substance abuse, it is also important to recognize that insight is not an all-or-nothing phenomenon; some people have complete insight into every aspect of their illness while others have only a glimmer. For example, Vicky had this to say when I interviewed her in the hospital shortly after her admission to receive treatment for a manic episode.

"I am emotionally unstable. I know I lose it sometimes. I get too grandiose and I have to be careful when I get on a roll. But that's just because I am creative."

"Is that what your family thinks?" I asked, knowing that her husband had practically dragged her into the hospital.

"My family thinks I'm bipolar and need to take lithium."

"What do you think?"

"It's possible that I do, but I don't know."

Even Matt showed a little bit of insight during the interview excerpted earlier when he told me, "Sometimes I get really paranoid. It's my nerves."

A glimmer of insight is an open door to making changes. Regardless of which aspects of insight are being measured, most studies find that the more aware a seriously mentally ill person is of his illness and of the benefits of treatment, the better his prognosis. Patients with better insight have shorter periods in a hospital and have fewer hospitalizations overall. No one knows for sure why this is the case, but it's easy to imagine, especially in light of studies showing that various kinds of insight into illness promote adherence to (involvement in) treatment. In the work conducted at our research center, we found that awareness of the beneficial effects of medication is one of the best predictors of adherence to medication.

In the case of psychiatric disorders, many people believe that side effects—not lack of insight—are the most important reason so many people refuse to take medication. As it turns out, side effects play a very small role in treatment refusal while poor insight is the biggest predictor of who will refuse to take medicine.

This research finding has been replicated many times over. Side effects are important, but their role in poor adherence is over-estimated. I believe this is true because so many people with poor insight give up trying to convince their doctors and loved ones that they are not sick and instead talk about side effects because they know they will be listened to. In a way, they do the reverse of what I will teach you in Part II of this book. Mentally ill persons with poor insight learn to speak the *doctor's* language and focus on those things the doctors (and, by extension, relatives) want to talk about.

Other forms of treatment adherence are similarly affected by poor insight. For example, Dr. Paul Lysaker and Dr. Morris

Bell of Yale University evaluated schizophrenia patients who were stabilized and enrolled in an outpatient work-rehabilitation program. Those who lacked insight had very poor adherence to the psychosocial treatments (day hospital programs, occupational therapy, etc.) in which they had agreed to participate, despite a stated desire to work. The researchers concluded that individuals with poor insight are likely to have more problems remaining in a course of treatment regardless of whether it involves drugs or psychotherapy.

Another myth is that the sicker one is, the worse the insight. Most studies find that this is not true. If left unattended, the level of insight is generally stable in most patients—those with poor insight while in crisis have lower levels of insight even when stable. Whether their symptoms are under control or not, they persist in the belief that they really don't need treatment. They may acknowledge that they were sick in the past, but do not in the present moment.

I am hopeful that, as the scientific community continues to turn its attention to this very serious problem, drug treatments for poor insight will improve.

In a study conducted by Dr. Joseph McEvoy and his colleagues at Duke University, patients with schizophrenia were followed from two-and-a-half to three-and-a-half years after discharge from the hospital. Although symptoms of psychosis improved in nearly all the patients over the course of their hospitalization, those who had been involuntarily committed did not show any improvement in level of insight into their illness. Furthermore, this low level of insight persisted throughout the follow-up period.

Not surprisingly, these same patients were more likely to be involuntarily committed over the course of follow-up. The authors concluded that an inability to see oneself as ill seems to be a persistent trait in many patients with schizophrenia and one that leads to commitment.

I agree with Dr. McEvoy. I have reviewed the literature, and most studies, with only a handful of exceptions, concur. However, this does not mean we should give up hope that medication may help with insight. There is new evidence about which I will tell you in Chapter 11 that shows promise and bears further investigation. I am hopeful, as the scientific community continues to turn its attention to this very serious problem, that drug treatments for poor insight will improve.

The last myth proved false by recent research concerns the idea that when one is seriously mentally ill, insight into illness leads to demoralization, depression, and suicidal thoughts. Having said that, suicide is clearly a very serious problem in both depression and schizophrenia, as estimates are that as many as one out of every ten persons with schizophrenia will die from suicide.

However, like most clinicians, I was taught that poor insight in patients with chronic mental illness, though problematic for treatment adherence, might be a Godsend with respect to suicide prevention. The assumption was that patients who don't understand that they're ill are less likely to become depressed and suicidal and that, alternatively, those patients who recognize illness will be more suicidal.

In fact, however, in a study my colleagues and I conducted, we found that awareness of having an illness was *not* associated with increased suicidal thoughts or behavior. This study suggests that poor insight is not a protective factor, as previously believed, and argues against the strategy of allowing patients who are unaware of their illness and refuse treatment simply to fend for themselves.

During my graduate training, I was also taught that when grandiose delusions (e.g., "I am married to someone rich and famous") are successfully treated, the risk of suicide increases. Anna-Lisa's mother, whom I mentioned in Chapter 1, had a delusion that the late-night talk show host David Letterman was her husband. When Anna-Lisa's mother died from suicide, it was after a prolonged involuntary hospitalization during which time she was medicated and her symptoms improved somewhat. Her mother's close friends believed that she had committed suicide because the medication had caused her to lose the fantasy world created by her delusions. In other words, when confronted with the reality that she was *not* the person her illness led her to believe she was, she couldn't bear it.

This is a terrible and all-too-common myth, because in reality, it wasn't insight or the loss of her delusions that led Anna-Lisa's mother to suicide; it was the fact that she didn't receive adequate follow-up treatment—she was not working closely with a doctor or therapist she trusted. Had there been someone to help guide her through her new-found grasp on reality, it is unlikely that she would have lost hope and taken her own life. The need for proper follow-up with a trusted mental health professional cannot be over-emphasized.

In Summary

The relevant facts revealed by research are that higher levels of insight into illness predict:

- reliable and consistent adherence to medication.
- fewer hospitalizations.
- shorter hospital stays.
- fewer commitments to the hospital.
- active involvement in all aspects of treatment.

Research also demonstrates the value of examining various aspects of insight independently. We now know that general insight into having an illness is far less important than insight into certain of its early warning signs and the beneficial effects of treatment.

In order to help your loved one, you will first need to understand the root of the problem. As you will learn in the next chapter, the research suggests that poor insight demonstrated by people with serious mental illness usually has little to do with being defensive, stubborn, uneducated, uncooperative or simply difficult.

3

The Root of the Problem:
New Research on Anosognosia
(Ã-nõ'sog-nõ'sê-ã)

"This is not surprising, since the brain, the same organ we use to think about ourselves and assess our needs, is the same organ that is affected in schizophrenia and bipolar disorder."

E. Fuller Torrey, commenting on the high prevalence of poor insight in persons with serious mental illness.

(*Schizophrenia and Manic Depressive Disorder*, 1996, page 27)

Sitting around the table with me were two nurses, a therapy aide, a social worker and a psychiatrist. We were in the middle of our weekly clinical team meeting discussing whether we thought Matt was well enough to be discharged from the hospital.

"His symptoms have vastly improved," began Maria, his primary nurse. "The hallucinations have responded to the medication. He's calmer and no longer paranoid."

"Both his mother and father are ready to have him come home again," added Cynthia, Matt's social worker, "and Dr. Remmers has agreed to see him as an outpatient."

"Sounds like we've got all our ducks lined up in a row." Dr. Preston, the team leader, capped the discussion and scribbled a note in Matt's medical chart.

"Only one thing troubles me," Cynthia interjected hesitantly. "I don't think he's going to follow through with the treatment plan. He still doesn't think there's anything wrong with him."

"He's taking his medication," I observed.

"For now. But he's really stubborn and so defensive. I don't think that will last more than a week or two after he hits the sidewalk."

I had to agree with Cynthia's prediction, but I didn't share her view as to *why* he wouldn't take his medication on the outside.

"What makes you say he's defensive?"

Nearly everyone around the table burst out laughing, thinking I was being facetious. "No, really, I'm serious," I said.

Dr. Brian Greene, the resident assigned to the case, jumped into the discussion.

"Well, he doesn't think there's anything wrong with him. As far as Matt's concerned, the only reason he's here is because his mother forced him into it. The man is full of pride and just plain stubborn. Don't get me wrong—I like him, but I don't think there's anything else we can do for him as long as he's in denial. No one's going to convince him that he's sick. He's just going to have to learn the lesson the hard way. He'll be back before he knows what hit him."

Dr. Preston, recognizing that Matt's discharge was a forgone conclusion, ended the discussion. "You're probably right about that and about the fact that there's nothing more we can offer him here. When he's ready to stop denying his problems, we can help. Until then, our hands are tied. Brian, you're meeting with Matt and his parents at three o'clock to go over the plan. Any questions?" After a moment's silence, Matt's medical chart was passed around the table for each of us to sign off on the discharge plan.

"All I need to do is get a job. There's nothing wrong with me."

During the first few years of my brother's illness (before I went to graduate school to become a clinical psychologist), I often thought he was being immature and stubborn. Asked about what his plans were after being discharged from yet another hospitalization, he ritually answered, "All I need to do is get a job. There's nothing wrong with me." His other stock answer was, "I am going to get married." Both desires were natural and understandable—but unrealistic given his recent history, the severity of the illness, and his refusal to accept treatment. Someday, perhaps, he would realize his desires, but it was very unlikely unless he was actively involved in the treatment recommended by his doctors.

It was exasperating to talk to Henry about why he wasn't taking his medication. Having limited experience with the illness, the only reason that I could think of for his adamant refusal was that he was being stubborn, defensive, and—to be frank—a pain in the rear. I was lucky that I thought of my brother only as being stubborn because, like many children of people with serious mental illness, Anna-Lisa often wondered if her mother didn't love her enough to want to get better. It took her mother's suicide to educate Anna-Lisa about what was really happening. And, for myself, it was only after I started working in the field and met many more people with serious mental illness that I stopped giving such theories much credence. It just never made sense to me that the pervasive unawareness and odd explanations given by people like Matt and my brother could be explained simply as having an immature personality or a lack of love.

You don't have to take my word for it. Let's look at the research for a more objective answer to the question of what causes poor insight and refusal to accept treatment.

Research on the Causes of Poor Insight

I have considered three possible causes of poor insight in the seriously mentally ill. First, it could stem from *defensiveness* — after all, it makes sense that someone who is seriously ill would be in denial about all the potential and promise for the future that has been taken by the disease.

Or, perhaps it's simply the result of *cultural or educational differences between the mentally ill person and the people who are trying to help him.* Differences in subculture and values are often blamed. For example, Anna-Lisa always believed that her mother's poor insight wasn't denial so much as a preference for the interesting and fantastic world her illness provided her. When she was symptomatic, the world was a magical place filled with adventures to be had and mysteries to explore. As a result, Anna-Lisa never wanted to question her mother's delusions, because she feared that by talking about them, she might take them away and somehow cause her mother even more pain.

The third possible cause is that poor insight into the illness stems from *the same brain dysfunction that is responsible for other symptoms of the disorder.* Historically, psychoanalytic theories predominated to explain poor insight in schizophrenia. The literature is rich with case studies suggesting that poor insight stems from defensive denial, but the question had never been tested in controlled studies until recently.

―――――――――――――――――――――――――――――――――――

Everyday defensiveness is not responsible for the gross deficits in insight that are so common in these patients.

―――――――――――――――――――――――――――――――――――

Two of my doctoral students, Chrysoula Kasapis and Elizabeth Nelson, took different approaches to this question in their thesis research. Dr. Kasapis examined the overall level of defensiveness in the patients she studied, while Dr. Nelson looked at the issue of stigma.

Neither approach to the question found anything of significance. Highly defensive patients were generally no more likely to have poor insight than those with little or no defensiveness. Similarly, how stigmatizing patients perceived their symptoms to be had little effect on insight into their illnesses. Everyone gets defensive from time to time and some are more prone to denial than others — the same holds true for people with serious mental illness. However, "everyday" defensiveness is not responsible for the gross deficits in insight that are so common in these patients.

Cultural differences between the examiner and patient may also play a role in the mislabeling of someone as having poor insight. In other words, a patient may be well aware of most, if not all, aspects of his mental illness, but his subculture might label it something else. Consequently, he would not use the label "mental illness" to describe himself. He might say instead, "I have a nervous problem," or, in the case of religious beliefs such as those common to some Caribbean countries, "I am possessed by evil spirits." The subculture of the afflicted person needs to be considered in any study of insight.

It's ironic, but many patients with poor insight into their own illnesses are excellent at diagnosing the same illness in others!

Related to the issue of cultural influences is the question of patient education. Has the patient ever been told that he or she has an illness? If so, has he or she been taught how to identify and label symptoms of the disorder? In my experience, most patients with poor insight have been told about the illness they have, yet either claim they haven't been told or adamantly disagree, claiming that their knowledge is superior to that of the doctors making the diagnosis. It's ironic, but many patients with poor insight into their own illnesses are excellent at diagnosing the same illness in others!

The answer to the question of whether half of all people with serious mental illness don't know they are ill because they have no information about the illness is actually obvious when you step back for a moment. If you had heartburn that was bad enough for a friend or relative to convince you to see your family doctor, who then diagnosed the problem as heart disease and explained that the pain was angina, you would stop referring to the pain as heartburn and start calling it angina. You would respond by making an appointment with a cardiologist and canceling your next visit with the gastroenterologist.

Why, then, do so many people with schizophrenia and bipolar disorder fail to do this? Why do they persist in calling their pain "heartburn" despite all evidence to the contrary?

A Concept of Self that is Stranded in Time

In our paper published in 1991, my colleagues and I proposed that poor insight in people with serious mental disorders is a consequence of, to coin a phrase, "a broken brain." We came to believe that pervasive lack of insight and the accompanying illogical ideas offered to explain being hospitalized stemmed from neurological deficits. At that time, we hadn't yet considered a neurological hypothesis to explain poor insight in bipolar disorder, but we felt there was good reason to believe that what we were seeing in patients with schizophrenia was a consequence of brain dysfunction rather than stubbornness, defensiveness, or ignorance about mental illness in general. The fact is that the brain circuitry responsible for recording and updating self-concept is not working properly in such patients.

For instance, *my* self-concept includes the following beliefs about my abilities: I can hold down a job; if I went back to school, I would be a competent student; I have the education and experience to be a therapist; and I am generally socially appropriate when I interact with others.

What are some of the beliefs you hold about yourself and your abilities? Do you believe that you can hold down a job? What if I told you that you were wrong, that you were incapable of working and might never find employment unless you swallowed some pills I had for you? And that you would have to take those pills for a very long time, possibly for the rest of your life?

What would you say to that? Probably the same thing my brother once said to me when I told him he would never hold down a job again unless he took his medication faithfully: "You're out of your mind!"

You would likely think I was joking, and after I convinced you that I was dead serious, you would come to believe I was crazy. After all, you *know* you can work—it's an obvious fact to you. And, if I involved other people, including relatives and doctors, you might start to feel persecuted and frightened.

That is *exactly* the experience of many with serious mental illness whom I have interviewed. Their neuropsychological deficits have left their concepts of self—their beliefs about what they can and cannot do—literally stranded in time. They believe they have all the same abilities and the same prospects they enjoyed prior to the onset of their illnesses. That's why we hear such unrealistic plans for the future from our loved ones.

If a Man Can Mistake his Wife for a Hat...

If you have never talked to someone who has suffered a stroke, brain tumor, or head injury, what I have just said might seem difficult to believe. If so, I recommend that you read *The Man Who Mistook His Wife for a Hat*, written by the late neurologist Oliver Sacks (also the author of the book upon which the movie "Awakenings" was based). Dr. Sacks had the gift of being able to describe, in vivid detail, the inner life of people who have suffered brain damage.

Writing about the case which gave title to his book, Dr. Sacks described a man who had cancer in the visual parts of his brain and noted that when he first met Dr. P., this music professor couldn't explain why he'd been referred to the clinic for an evaluation. He appeared normal—there was nothing unusual about his speech—and he displayed high intelligence. As the neurological evaluation proceeded, however, bizarre perceptions emerged. When asked to put his shoes back on, he delayed—gazing at his foot with intense but misplaced concentration. When Dr. Sacks asked if he could help, Dr. P. declined the offer and continued looking around. Finally, he grabbed his foot and asked, "This is my shoe, no?" When shown where his shoe actually was, he replied, "I thought that was my foot."

There was nothing at all wrong with Dr. P.'s vision—it was the way his brain was constructing and categorizing his perceptions that was disturbed. Later, when he was sitting with his wife in Dr. Sacks's office, he thought it was time to leave and reached for his hat. But instead of his hat, he grabbed his wife's head and tried to lift it off. He had apparently mistaken his wife's head for a hat! When giving talks about poor insight in serious mental disorders, I often like to say, "If brain damage can cause a man to mistake his wife for a hat, it is easy to imagine how it can cause someone to mistake his *past self* for his *current self.*"

In the late 1980s, I worked extensively with neurological patients, administering psychological tests designed to uncover the deficits caused by their brain damage. I couldn't help noticing the similarities between the neurological syndrome called *anosognosia* (i.e., unawareness of deficits, symptoms, or signs of illness) and poor insight in persons with serious mental illness. Anosognosia bears a striking resemblance to the type of poor insight we have been discussing. This resemblance includes both symptomatic and neurological similarities.

For example, patients with anosognosia will frequently give strange explanations, or what neurologists call *confabulations*, to explain any observations that contradict their beliefs that they are not ill. One 42-year-old man I evaluated had been in a car accident and had suffered a serious head injury that damaged tissue in the right frontal, parietal, and temporal lobes of his brain, leaving him paralyzed on the left side of his body. When I met with him about a week after the accident, I asked if he could raise his left arm for me and he answered "yes." When I asked him to do it, he lay there expressionless, unable to move his paralyzed arm. I pointed out that he had not moved his arm. He disagreed. So, I asked him to do it again while looking at his arm. When he saw that he could not move his arm, he became flustered. I asked him why he did not move it, and he refused to answer at first. When I pressed him, he said, "I know this is going to sound crazy, but you must have tied it down or something."

Anosognosia has been with us for as long as our species has enjoyed the benefits of consciousness. More than 2,000 years ago, L.A. Seneca, writing on the moral implications of self-beliefs, described what appears to be a case of anosognosia following hemianopia (blindness caused by brain damage): "*Incredible as it might appear...She does not know that she is blind. Therefore, again and again, she asks her guardian to take her elsewhere. She claims that my home is dark.*" How could someone not realize she was blind? And why, when faced with the evidence, would she seek to explain away the blindness?

When one's conception of who one is gets stranded in time, one can't help ignoring or explaining away any evidence that contradicts it.

The man who had been paralyzed in the car accident could not understand that he could no longer move the left side of his body.

It didn't fit with what he believed about himself (that his arm and leg worked fine), so he couldn't help trying to explain away any evidence to the contrary. He was just like the blind woman who did not understand that she was blind—and more easily believed an alternative explanation than the truth (e.g., the house was dark). Every day, someone with a serious mental illness utters similar explanations to buttress his belief that there is nothing wrong with him. When one's conception of who one is gets stranded in time, cut off from important new information, one can't help ignoring or explaining away any evidence that contradicts it. As a result, many chronically mentally ill persons attribute their hospitalizations to fights with parents, misunderstandings, etc. Like neurological patients with anosognosia, they appear rigid in their unawareness, unable to integrate new information that is contrary to their erroneous beliefs.

One final similarity between neurological patients with anosognosia and the seriously mentally ill involves the patch-like pattern of poor insight. Pockets of unawareness and awareness often coexist side by side. For example, the anosognosia patient may be aware of a memory deficit but unaware of paralysis. Similarly, we have seen many patients with schizophrenia who are aware of particular symptoms while remaining completely unaware of others.

Damage to particular brain areas can result in anosognosia. Studies of anosognosia, therefore, provide a practical starting point for hypothesizing about the brain structures responsible for insight in persons with serious mental disorders. Neurological patients with anosognosia are frequently found to have lesions (i.e., damage of one kind or another) to the frontal lobes of their brains. Interestingly, research has shown that these same areas of the brain are often dysfunctional in people with serious mental illness.

In one study of neurological patients at Hillside Hospital in Queens, New York, conducted in collaboration with Dr. William

Barr and Dr. Alexandra Economou, I compared patterns of unawareness in three groups of patients suffering damage to three different regions of the brain. This study was funded by the Stanley Foundation and had as one of its goals identifying the brain dysfunction most likely to produce awareness deficits. As expected, patients with frontal lesions were more likely to show problems with insight into their illnesses than patients with left posterior damage. Let's look at an example.

George, a 71-year-old man who had suffered a stroke, was asked to draw the clock on the left side of the figure that appears below. Before drawing the clock, he was asked, "Do you think you will have any difficulty copying this picture?"

George was instructed to use the following 4-point scale to answer the question: 0 = no difficulty, 1 = some difficulty, 2 = much difficulty, and 3 = cannot do. He answered "0" and said he would have no difficulty. The right side of the figure shows the drawing he made after exerting great effort.

More striking than his inability to recognize that the stroke had left him unable to perform such a simple task was what happened next. When asked if he'd had any difficulty drawing the clock, he answered, "No, not at all." Further questioning revealed that he could not see or comprehend the differences between his clock and ours.

When it was pointed out to him that his numbers drifted past the circle, he became flustered and said, "Wait, that can't be my drawing. What happened to the one I drew? You switched it on me!" This is an example of a *confabulation*. Confabulations are the product of a brain "reflex" that fills in gaps in our understanding and memory of the world around us. Almost everyone confabulates a little — you've heard people stop in the middle of recounting something that happened to them and say something like, "Wait, I was lying. I don't know why I said that. It didn't happen that way!" This is an example of an instance when someone realizes he has confabulated and corrects himself.

Confabulations are "constructed" memories and/or experiences that are especially common in people with brain dysfunction. However, in such individuals, we don't usually observe self-correction, because they don't understand the need for correction. George wasn't lying when he said I had switched the drawing on him. It was the only thing that made any sense to him, so for a moment, he believed that was what had happened.

He was operating under beliefs that were linked to his past self rather than his current self.

In his book *The Principles of Psychology*, William James wrote: "Whilst part of what we perceive comes through our senses from the object before us, another part (and it may be the larger part) always comes from our own mind."

There are few better examples of James's insight than the one I have just given you. George "saw" his drawing using his sense of vision. But his *perception* of the clock — the image of the drawing that was processed in his brain — was something altogether different from what his eyes saw. George had a concept of himself, a *self-schema,* that included the belief that he could easily copy a simple drawing of a clock.

You have the same belief as part of your self-schema. You might not consider yourself artistically endowed, but you believe that you could produce a reasonable facsimile of the drawing if asked to. In a sense, this belief was stranded in George's brain, disconnected from his visual senses and left unmodified by the stroke he had suffered. He was operating under beliefs that were linked to his *past self* rather than his *current self*. He *saw* the numbers drifting outside his lopsided circle, but he *perceived* the numbers to be in their proper place inside a symmetrical circle. Our brains are built to order, and even help construct, our perceptions.

Here is a simple example of what I am talking about. Answer this question: What letter appears in the box you see to the right?

If you answered "E" you saw what the majority of people who are given this task see. But in reality, you did not *see* the letter E. What you saw is a line with two right angles (a box-like version of the letter "C") and a short line that is unconnected to the longer one. You likely answered "E" because you *perceived* the letter E. The visual processing and memory circuits of your brain "closed the gap" between the lines so you could answer the question.

To prove that poor insight in serious mental disorders is neurologically based, however, my colleagues and I needed more than observed similarities with neurological patients. We needed testable hypotheses and data that were confirmatory.

Knowing that patients with schizophrenia frequently show poor performance on neuropsychological tests of frontal lobe function, we hypothesized that there should be a strong correlation between various aspects of unawareness of illness and performance on those tests.

Dr. Donald Young and his colleagues in Toronto, Canada, quickly tested and confirmed our hypothesis. They studied patients with schizophrenia to examine whether performance on neuropsychological tests of frontal lobe function predicted the level of insight into illness, and the result showed a strong association between the two. Of particular note is the fact that this correlation was independent of other cognitive functions they tested, including overall IQ. In other words, poor insight was related to dysfunction of the frontal lobes of the brain rather than to a more generalized problem with intellectual functioning. Taken together, these results strongly support the idea that poor insight into illness and resulting treatment refusal stem from a mental defect rather than informed choice.

But just as one swallow does not make a summer, one research finding does not make an indisputable fact. The next step in determining more definitively whether poor insight into illness is a consequence of frontal lobe dysfunction is to replicate the findings of Young and his colleagues in a new group of patients.

As it turns out, the finding that poorer insight is significantly correlated with frontal lobe dysfunction (and reduced grey matter in the frontal lobes) has been replicated many times by various research groups (see table below). The list of replications I give here will undoubtedly be added to by the time you read these words.

Repeated replications by independent researchers are infrequent in psychiatric research, so the fact that various researchers have found essentially the same thing as Young and his colleagues speaks to the strength of the relationship between insight and the frontal lobes of the brain. A few studies have not found this relationship, but in those cases methodological flaws in the design of the research are likely the reason.

Executive (Frontal) Dysfunction and Poor Insight

- Young et al. *Schizophrenia Research,* 1993
- Lysaker et al. *Psychiatry,* 1994
- Kasapis et al. *Schizophrenia Research,* 1996
- McEvoy et al. *Schizophrenia Bulletin,* 1996
- Voruganti et al. *Canadian Journal of Psychiatry,* 1997
- Lysaker et al. *Acta Psychiatr Scand,* 1998
- Young et al. *Journal of Nervous and Mental Disease,* 1998
- Bell et al. Chapter in: *Insight & Psychosis,* Amador & David, Eds. 1998
- Morgan et al. *Schizophrenia Research,* 1999a & 1999b
- Smith et al. *Journal of Nervous and Mental Disease,* 1999
- Smith et al. *Schizophrenia Bulletin,* 2000
- Laroi et al. *Psychiatry Research,* 2000
- Bucklet et al. *Comprehensive Psychiatry,* 2001
- Lysaker et al. *Schizophrenia Research,* 2003
- Drake et al. *Schizophrenia Research,* 2003
- Morgan and David (review) in *Insight and Psychosis,* 2nd Edition (Oxford University Press, 2004)
- Keshavan et al. *Schizophrenia Research,* 2004
- Aleman et al. *British Journal of Psychiatry,* 2006
- Pia & Tamietto, *European Archives of Psychiatry and Clinical Neuroscience,* 2006
- Shad et al., *Schizophrenia Research,* 2006
- Sartory et al. *Schizophrenia Bulletin,* 2009
- Bora *Schizophrenia Research,* 2017
- Asmal et al. *Schizophrenia Research,* 2017

Anatomical Brain Differences and Poor Insight

There is also an emerging body of literature linking poor insight in schizophrenia and other psychotic illnesses to functional and structural abnormalities in the brain, usually involving the frontal lobes (e.g., the Asmal et al. study above). For example, evidence from brain imaging and post-mortem studies find differences in the brains of schizophrenia patients who have insight or awareness of illness, when compared to those who do not.

From 1992 to 2017, 22 studies compared the brains of individuals with schizophrenia, with and without awareness of illness. All but two studies found significant differences (between aware and unaware subjects) in one or more anatomical structures. A variety of anatomical structures were involved — including the anterior insula, anterior cingulate cortex, medial frontal cortex, and inferior parietal cortex. Three of the above studies included individuals with schizophrenia who had never been treated with medication, discounting the hypothesis that these brain differences resulted from treatment. A more detailed review of these and other brain-imaging studies (e.g., using MRI, CT and PET scans) can be found in *Insight and Psychosis*, Amador XF and David AS (Editors), Oxford University Press, 2005.

The research discussed above and other newer studies that link poor insight to structural brain abnormalities lead us to only one conclusion. In most patients with schizophrenia and related psychotic disorders, deficits in insight and resulting non-adherence to treatment stem from a broken brain rather than stubbornness or denial.

Anosognosia and our Authoritative Diagnostic Manuals (i.e., the DSMs)

If you are dealing with a mental health professional who is holding on to the outdated idea that severe and persistent problems with insight are a consequence of "denial" (i.e., a coping mechanism), ask him or her to look at the "Schizophrenia and Related Disorders" section of the *DSM-IV-TR*. This is the grey-colored DSM most clinicians have. Ask them to read page 304:

Associated Features and Disorders

"A majority of individuals with Schizophrenia have poor insight regarding the fact that they have a psychotic illness. Evidence suggests that poor insight is a manifestation of the illness itself rather than a coping strategy... comparable to the lack of awareness of neurological deficits seen in stroke, termed anosognosia."

Now, if the person you are trying to educate is extremely resistant and a careful reader, he or she may say something like, "Yes, but I also see that Dr. Amador was the co-chair of this section of the *DSM*, so he just wrote what he already believes. It doesn't prove anything!"

If that happens, have the person read the introduction to this revision. He will learn that every sentence in this version of the *DSM* had to be *peer-reviewed* before it was added. Peer review in this context involved other experts in the field receiving the proposed text along with all the research articles that supported the changes my co-chair and I wanted to make. *All changes had to be supported by reliable and valid research findings.*

So, although the field has been slow to give up outdated theories about poor insight in these disorders (thinking it's denial rather than anosognosia), we are making progress.

But what about the most recent edition of the DSM published in 2013? This is the copy (purple cover) of the DSM currently in widespread use. Here is what the DSM 5 has to say about "poor insight" in schizophrenia (on page 101):

Associated Features and Disorders

"Unawareness of illness is typically a symptom rather than a coping strategy. It is comparable to the lack of awareness of neurological deficits following brain damage, termed anosognosia... This symptom is the most common predictor of

nonadherence to treatment. It has been found to predict higher relapse rates, increased number of involuntary treatments, poorer psychosocial functioning, aggression, and a poorer course of illness.

Anosognosia versus Denial

Often, I am asked the question: "How can I know whether I am dealing with anosognosia versus denial?" There are three main things you should look for:

1. The lack of insight is severe and persistent (it lasts for months or years).
2. The beliefs ("I am not sick," "I don't have any symptoms," etc.) are fixed and do not change even after the person is confronted with overwhelming evidence that they are wrong.
3. Illogical explanations, or confabulations, that attempt to explain away the evidence of illness are common.

Ideally, you would also want to know if neuropsychological testing revealed executive dysfunction. But regardless of whether the problem is neurologically based or stems from intractable defensiveness, or both, the most important question is: How can you help this person to accept treatment? That is the focus of the rest of this book.

The cause of the severe and persistent "denial" may be less important than how you choose to deal with it.

Remember, the cause of the severe and persistent "denial" may be less important than how you choose to deal with it. The fact that the person you're helping does not see what you see and, his or her belief cannot be changed, is all you need to know to move forward.

Part II

How to Help Using LEAP

"You can't always get what you want.
But if you try sometime,
you just might find,
you get what you need!"

— Mick Jagger and Keith Richards —
The Rolling Stones, *Let it Bleed,* 1969

4

The Right and Wrong Approach

"Tell me one last thing," said Harry. "Is this real? Or has this been happening in my head?"

Dumbledore beamed at him... "Of course, it is happening in your head, Harry, but why on earth should that mean it is not real?"

—J.K. Rowling—
Harry Potter and the Deathly Hallows, 2007

Dr. Karen Holloway sighed and said, "Michael's back," as she walked toward where I was sitting in the nurse's station. "I need you to go to the ER and do his admission," she added.

"Michael Kass?" I asked, incredulous.

"Afraid so," Karen replied, a bit amused by my surprise. "Get used to it, Xavier. Some patients are stuck in the revolving door, and Michael's one of them."

This was 1988 and Karen was the chief resident at the hospital in New York City where I was an intern. To this day, she remains one of the more compassionate, bright and level-headed clinicians with whom I have ever had the pleasure of working. The diagnosis of "Revolving Door Patient" was not one she made lightly or without compassion.

Michael Kass had been discharged from the hospital only six weeks earlier after a one-month hospitalization. When he left, he was no longer hearing voices. His delusions still lingered, but he felt little pressure to talk about them and he was scheduled to receive follow-up treatment in one of our outpatient clinics.

Judging by Karen's comment, I guess I hadn't hidden my disappointment and surprise that he was back so soon. I took the stairs two at a time, eight floors down, to the Emergency Room — no use waiting for the overburdened elevators — and walked to the door labeled "Psych ER." Behind this door, sequestered from the rest of the ER service, was a suite of five rooms with four patient bays to the left and the nurses' station to the right. As I entered, I took a quick right and ducked into the nurses' station — I didn't want Michael to know I was there until I'd had a chance to talk to the triage nurse. The report I got was frustrating to hear.

After leaving the hospital, Michael had gone home to live with his parents but had not shown up for his first outpatient appointment. His parents, in their late sixties, hadn't known that Michael hadn't gone to see his doctor. They'd asked about his appointment, but he hadn't wanted to talk about it. They'd called the clinic, but no one would tell them whether or not their 35-year-old son had kept his doctor's appointment. They also hadn't known that after the one-week supply of medications he'd been given when leaving the hospital had run out, he'd never had the prescription refilled.

I spent about twenty minutes looking at his old chart, which the triage nurse had ordered up from medical records. Then I stepped out of the nurses' station and greeted my new-old patient.

"Hi, Michael, how are you?"

"Dr. Amadorafloor! What are *you* doing here?" he answered, *clanging*[1], laughing and talking a mile a minute. "You've got to

1 A feature of thought disorder, a frequent symptom of psychosis, that involves word associations based on rhyme.

get me out of here! I was minding my own business—I wasn't hurting anyone—and the police got it all wrong. Get me out of here, okay? You've got to get me out because..."

I tried to interrupt. "Michael, Michael, hold on, wait up a minute!"

"I'm not supposed to be here. They'll find me here if I stay. Gotta go, gotta get out, okay?"

"Michael, try to slow down and tell me what happened."

"I'm telling you what happened. I'm not supposed to be here," he shot back, clearly annoyed with me.

It took almost an hour to get through the checklist I was trained to use. I completed a *mental status exam*[2], evaluated his current symptoms, and listened to his version of what had happened and why he was in the Psych ER. Excusing myself while he was again pleading with me to get him out, I escaped to the nurses' station again to write down what I had learned.

Michael was once again hearing the voices of government agents who were commenting on his every move. While we were talking, I asked him what the voices were saying and he repeated, "He is sitting on the bed, talking with that doctor. He can't escape us now." Given the voices he was hearing, it isn't surprising he'd developed the delusion that some secret federal agency was monitoring his movements and planning to assassinate him.

I noted in his chart the re-emergence of the hallucinations and exacerbation of the longstanding delusion about government agents persecuting him. I also noted that he was not currently suicidal or homicidal, that his "insight into illness" was poor, and a number of other observations I had made while interviewing him. My written recommendation was to restart the antipsychotic medication he'd been on when he was discharged six weeks

---

2 A cornerstone of psychiatric assessment, the mental status exam involves an assessment of the clarity of consciousness, memory, attention, emotion, thought process, insight into illness, and various symptoms of mental illness.

before and to admit him to our inpatient psychiatric unit "for stabilization." Then I went back to see Michael, told him my recommendation, and asked him to sign himself into the hospital for a couple of weeks.

He refused. "The only thing wrong with me is that I'm going to get killed if I stay here any longer!" he said.

Since he had been found hiding in a subway train tunnel and had struggled with the police when they extracted him, I thought we had a fairly good case for an involuntary admission. When he was found, he hadn't eaten or bathed in several days and he had made camp dangerously close to an active track, explaining to police that "they [the federal agents] would never think to look for me here." I called Dr. Holloway and she agreed—the appropriate papers were signed to admit him against his will for 72 hours. If he didn't want to stay after the 72 hours, and if at that time we felt he was still a danger to himself because of his mental illness, we would take him before a mental health court and try to get a judge to order thirty days of involuntary treatment.

When I explained the plan to Michael, he understandably went ballistic. He was terribly frightened and felt certain that he would be killed if he stayed in the hospital. However, after accepting medication by injection, he calmed down considerably and was moved upstairs to the psychiatric ward.

Unless something was done to engage Michael in treatment, this hospitalization would be nothing more than a band-aid.

Though we had resolved the current crisis, unless something was done to engage Michael in treatment, this hospitalization would be nothing more than a band-aid. He would be "stabilized" and discharged with prescriptions he would never fill and an appointment he would never keep because, as he put it, "I am not sick! I don't need medicine—I need protection from the feds!"

The Wrong Approach

I was using the medical model with Michael, which in most cases is the wrong approach to take for dealing with the long-term issue of poor insight and refusal to take medicine. The medical model is supposed to work, more or less, in the following way:

Once the diagnosis and treatment are decided upon, the patient is informed of both. If the patient refuses, and if he fits the legal criteria for an involuntary admission to a hospital, the doctors take charge. In some cases, medical doctors operating under a benevolent paternal ethic are able to order treatment against a person's wishes. Like a parent who knows what's best for her child, the physician can take control by admitting the person and treating him against his will. We abide by similar, though less dramatic laws every day (e.g., laws that require seatbelts, mandatory rabies inoculation of pets, motorcycle helmets, those that prohibit drunk driving).

My next task, under this model, was to educate Michael about his illness and the need for treatment. If you are reading this book, you know that when it comes to individuals like Michael, education about their illness does not translate into their gaining insight. And, indeed, Michael didn't gain insight over the two-week period he was in the hospital.

I told him all about delusions and hallucinations and confronted him about his "denial" of the illness. I explained to him the nature of the problems he had and why he should accept the treatment being offered. As during his previous hospitalization, once he became more stable, he readily agreed that he would take the medication when he left the hospital. When I told him I thought he was just saying that so he could get out of the hospital, he sometimes sheepishly admitted to the lie and told me there was nothing wrong with him except the fact that people wouldn't leave him alone. But most often he would stick to the "party line" and say, "I know the medication helps me and that I need to take it." Ironically, as some of his symptoms responded to the medication, he got better at consistently feigning allegiance to the doctor's orders.

For people with serious mental illness who are also unaware of their illnesses, this traditional medical approach rarely works. It rests on the mistaken assumption that the patient has come to see the doctor because he feels he has a problem and wants help. It assumes a collaborative approach from the start—the doctor as an ally, not an adversary.

Although the details might differ, Michael's story of hospitalization followed by outpatient noncompliance, worsening illness, and readmission to the hospital...is all too typical. So was my inadequate response to the bigger problem of what would happen to him when we were done with him (again). I was operating under a medical model that focused on the tasks of diagnosis and treatment. This is the wrong approach when dealing with someone who has, for many years, consistently argued that there is nothing wrong with him and doesn't need help. It's not a bad approach for the short term, but it's mostly worthless over the long term because the "patient" doesn't *see* himself as a patient.

||||||||||||||||||||||||||||||||||||||||||||||||||||||||||||||||||||||||||||||||||||||||||||||||||||||||||||||||||||||||||||||||||||||||

If you can imagine something like this happening to you, then you have some idea of what it is like for someone with a mental illness to have a delusion and anosognosia.

||||||||||||||||||||||||||||||||||||||||||||||||||||||||||||||||||||||||||||||||||||||||||||||||||||||||||||||||||||||||||||||||||||||||

Imagine I told you that you did not live where you live. You might laugh and tell me to stop joking around. But what if I produced a restraining order from a court that ordered you to stay away from what you told me was your home address?

Taking it further, let's say you live with other people, perhaps members of your family, and you saw that they had signed off on this court order. What would you think? Then, imagine that you then called them to ask why they'd signed off and they said something like, "You seem like a nice person, but if you keep coming around here we are going to call the police. You don't live here and we don't want to press charges, but we will if you put us in that position. Please stop calling us. You need help!"

If you can imagine something like this happening to you, then you have some idea of what it is like for someone with a mental illness to have a delusion and anosognosia.

Let's go a little further with the analogy. Imagine you went home only to be arrested by the police. The nice people at your address did not want to press charges, so the police took you to the ER. Would you be receptive to my advice that you should take psychiatric drugs for your "delusion" that you live where you *know* you live? I doubt it. I have done this role play countless times during training and the answer is always "No!" When I ask why, my role-play partner usually laughs and says, "Because it's the truth. I know who I am and where I live!"

That's what it's like for a person with a serious mental illness to have a delusion *and* anosognosia. The medical model will not win this person's trust or cooperation. Like you or me in this situation, once the person is out of the hospital and on his own, he will *not* take medicine. If you can see the situation from that person's perspective, it makes sense, doesn't it?

The Right Approach

In my experience, it is often easy to change an adversarial relationship into an alliance and long-term engagement in treatment. It takes focused effort but isn't hard to do once you learn the main lessons. The hardest part is putting aside your preconceptions and remembering that no amount of arguing has previously changed your loved one's opinion.

My best advice to you is to stop trying to convince him he is ill. When you accept your powerlessness to convince him you know the answer to the penultimate question (is he, or is he not mentally ill), you will begin to open doors you didn't even know existed. Remember, if you had truly succeeded in convincing your loved one he has a mental illness, you would not be reading this book. The first step, therefore, is to stop arguing and start listening to your loved one in a way that leaves him feeling that his point of view — including his delusional ideas and the belief that he is not sick — is being respected.

The first step is to stop arguing and start listening to your loved one in a way that leaves him feeling that his point of view — including his delusional ideas and the belief that he is not sick — is being respected.

Professor Dumbledore's answer to Harry Potter's question, quoted at the start of this chapter, is exactly right. For all intents and purposes, your loved one's experience is very real indeed. To him, he is truly *not* sick.

If you can relate to your loved one in this way, you will be much closer to becoming his ally and working together to find the reasons *he* may have to accept treatment — even though he is not sick. You don't have to agree with his reality — the "realness" of his experience — but you *do* need to listen and *genuinely* respect it.

My colleagues and I have helped many patients accept treatment for a wide range of problems they feel have nothing to do with mental illness (e.g., to relieve the stress caused by the conspiracy against them; to help them sleep; to get their families "off their back"; to lower the volume on the voices being transmitted by the CIA). That said, the relationship we forged proved more important than any specific reason. Below, you will learn much more about the nature of the relationship that made all the difference.

Even so, I don't expect you to immediately embrace this idea.

Most people find it counterintuitive and even a little scary. Others like the concept of stepping back from the debate about whether or not the person is ill but are not sure about how it is going to help. Let me start addressing these concerns by describing my approach and the science behind it.

Motivational Enhancement Therapy and LEAP

Anyone who has dealt with denial in a loved one knows that it can't be fixed simply by educating the person about the problem he doesn't believe he has. Such attempts are futile because the "patient" doesn't see himself as a patient. And, research shows that confrontation and group "interventions" rarely work. In fact, contrary to what most people believe, "interventions" often do more harm than good!

So what *does* work? Motivational Enhancement Therapy (MET). It is a science-proven method that helps people in denial accept treatment. It was first developed more than 20 years ago for professionals like me who were working with substance- and alcohol-abusing patients. Unfortunately, despite its proven effectiveness for engaging people with substance abuse problems in treatment, few therapists are trained to use it with patients who have serious mental illnesses. This needs to change, as there is plenty of research to support using MET with such individuals.

In 2002, the *American Journal of Psychiatry* published a review by Dr. Annette Zygmunt and her colleagues of studies published over a 20-year period and aimed at improving medication adherence in schizophrenia. The researchers found that "although interventions and family therapy programs relying on psychoeducation were common in clinical practice, *they were typically ineffective* [with respect to improving adherence to treatment]...*Motivational techniques* [on the other hand] were common features of *successful programs*." By "motivational techniques," the authors meant the main elements of MET.

---

*I realized almost immediately that the specific
communication skills and strategies we were teaching therapists
could be learned by anyone.*

Relying on the same evidence base reviewed by Dr. Zygmunt and her colleagues, Dr. Aaron T. Beck (considered by many to be the "father" of cognitive psychology) and I developed a form of MET we called "Medication and Insight Therapy" (MAIT) for an inpatient research study to be used with people who have serious mental illness.

At the time (mid-1990s), we taught this method only to therapists. But I realized almost immediately that anyone could learn the specific communication skills and strategies we were teaching. I felt it was more a communication style than a complicated therapeutic intervention and came to believe that you don't need an M.D., M.S.W., or Ph.D. to use the main elements of this approach effectively. Consequently, I developed a lay-friendly version that can be taught to family members, individuals in law enforcement, and mental health professionals alike.

Listen-Empathize-Agree-Partner (LEAP) method

The result was the Listen-Empathize-Agree-Partner® (LEAP®) method. Over the past twenty years, since the publication of the first edition of this book, I have taught LEAP to tens of thousands of people across the country and overseas. Although the focus of my LEAP workshops was to show family members, health providers, and criminal justice professionals how to convince someone with serious mental illness to accept treatment, people at every seminar have commented on the usefulness of this method across a range of problems. That has been my experience as well.

So, whether you believe your loved one has anosognosia for mental illness, addiction, or simple denial of illness, LEAP can help.

5

Learning to LEAP

When I was five years old, I wanted to be Batman. It's true that Superman, Spiderman and the Hulk were also appealing, but for me, they were all a distant second to the "caped crusader." It wasn't his mask and ears, which I remember thinking looked goofy—it was that amazing "Bat Utility Belt." I had to have a Batman costume for Halloween—nothing else would do—and I still remember how I felt when I strapped on that belt for the first time. I had the power to do good—I could conquer all evil, set things right and live to tell the tale.

The best thing about Batman was that he was a regular person. He did not have superpowers—it was his tool belt that set him apart. There were many high-tech tools in his belt, but my favorite was the grappling hook, attached to a dental-floss-thin rope, that he used to walk up the sides of buildings. With those tools, there was no wall he could not climb, no obstacle he could not overcome. There was no enemy he could not defeat.

I want you to imagine that you, too, have a tool belt. It can be made of any material you like, stylish (Dolce and Gabbana) or purely functional (Craftsman). Imagine it is full on the left side with all the tools we use when relying on the medical and psycho-educational approaches (e.g., making a diagnosis, educating the person about his diagnosis, giving him his prognosis and prescriptions for treatment, reality testing about delusions). These tools are highly effective when we are dealing with persons who have insight and want our help—ideal for persons who identify themselves as patients or consumers.

Now, I want you to imagine that your tool belt is empty on the right side. Loops, hooks, and pockets all lay open and ready to receive the tools you will need to help someone accept treatment even though he does not believe he is ill. I'm going to provide you with the tools to fill that side of your belt. They will serve you well, but you'll have to practice using them.

The first and most important tool you will put in your belt is the focus of the next chapter—the *Reflective Listening Tool.* But you will also learn how not to "buy into delusions" while listening without judgment and how to *delay giving your opinion* when asked potential deal-breaker questions like, "So, do you think I'm sick and should take this medicine?" I will also explain all the reasons you should delay answering such questions and how to choose the right time to give your opinion. And I'll provide a tool for *giving your opinion* in a manner that allows your loved one to save face, retain dignity, not feel betrayed, and most importantly, *stay in the conversation and not walk away.*

To make all this happen you have to put your goal of convincing your loved one he is sick high up on a shelf, at least for the time being.

I think you will find that LEAP's effectiveness for dealing with someone in denial or with anosognosia is immediately intuitive. Once you learn the basic principles, it simply makes sense that it will work far better than what you've been doing all along. The core tools are *Listening* (using "reflective" listening), *Empathizing* (strategically—especially about those feelings you've ignored during your previous arguments about your loved one's being sick and needing treatment), *Agreeing* (on those things you can agree on and agreeing to disagree about the others), and ultimately *Partnering* (forming a partnership to achieve the goals you share).

More often than not, the first aim of LEAP is to repair the damage done to the relationship by your (or others) previously adhering to the medical model and taking the "doctor knows best approach."

The second very important task is to create a relationship in which your loved ones feel respected and not judged. This will help them find *their own reasons* to accept treatment. To make all this happen you have to put your goal of convincing your loved one he is sick high up on a shelf, at least for the time being.

If you balk at this advice take a moment to answer the following question: How many times have you told your loved one he or she needs treatment? Has it worked? This is a good time to recall Albert Einstein's definition of insanity: *Doing the same thing over and over again and expecting a different result.* Who's the insane person in this scenario?!

|||||||||||||||||||||||||||||||||||||||||||||||||||||||||||||||||||||||||||||||||||||||||||||||||||||||||||||||||||||||||||||||||||||||||||||||||||||||||||||||||||||||

Listen with only one goal: to understand the other person's point of view and reflect your understanding back to him without judgment.

|||||||||||||||||||||||||||||||||||||||||||||||||||||||||||||||||||||||||||||||||||||||||||||||||||||||||||||||||||||||||||||||||||||||||||||||||||||||||||||||||||||||

The cornerstone of LEAP is reflective listening. It is also the one feature of the method that immediately turns down the volume on everyone's anger, builds trust, and mends fences. The reason is that you listen with only one goal: *to understand the other person's point of view and reflect your understanding back to him without judgment.* You don't comment on what he said, point out ways in which you think he's wrong, judge, or react in any way. (Sounds easy until the person starts talking about the fact that there's absolutely nothing wrong and he doesn't need treatment!)

Listen

Reflective listening is a skill that needs to be cultivated — it doesn't come naturally to most people. To succeed, you will need to learn to really listen and not *react* to what your loved one feels, wants, and believes. Then, after you think you understand what you are told, you need to reflect to him or her, in your own words, your understanding of what you just heard.

The trick is to do this without commenting, disagreeing, or arguing. If you succeed, your loved one's resistance to talking with you about treatment will lessen and you will begin to gain a clear idea of *his* experience of the illness and the treatment he doesn't want. When you know how your loved one experiences the idea of having a mental illness, addiction and/or taking psychiatric drugs, you will have a foothold you can use to start moving forward. But you will also need to know what his hopes and expectations are for the future, *whether or not you believe they're realistic*. If you can reflect back an accurate understanding of these experiences, hopes, and expectations, your loved one is going to be much more open to talking with you. More importantly, he is going to be much more open to hearing what you have to say.

Empathize

The second tool for your tool belt involves learning *when* and *how* to express empathy. If there were a moral to each technique, the one for empathizing would go something like this: *If you want someone to seriously consider your point of view, be certain he feels you have seriously considered his. Quid pro quo.* That means you must empathize with all the reasons he has for not wanting to accept treatment, even those you think are "crazy." And you *especially* want to empathize with any feelings connected to delusions (such as fear, anger, or even elation, if the delusion is grandiose). But don't worry — empathizing with how a particular delusion makes one feel is *not* the same as agreeing that the belief is true. This may seem like a minor point, but, as you will learn, the right kind of empathy will make a tremendous difference in how receptive your loved one is to *your* concerns and opinions.

Agree

Find common ground and stake it out. Knowing that what *you want* for your loved one is something *he does not want* for himself can make it seem as if there *is* no common ground. You want him to admit he's sick and accept treatment. He doesn't think he's sick, so why in the world would he accept treatment for an illness he doesn't have? To avoid coming to an impasse, you need to look closer for common ground and for whatever motivation the other person may have for changing. Common ground always exists, even between the most extreme opposing positions.

One area you both can almost certainly agree upon is wanting the relationship to be conflict-free, wanting the relationship to be better.

The emphasis here is on acknowledging that your loved one has personal choice and responsibility for the decisions he makes about his life. When you use the *Agreement Tool*, you become a neutral observer, pointing out the various things you *do* agree upon. If invited, you can also point out the positive and negative consequences of decisions your loved one has made. That means refraining from saying things like, "See, if you had taken your medication, you wouldn't have ended up in the hospital." Or, "If you hadn't been high, you would not be in the trouble you're in." Your focus is on *making observations together* – identifying facts upon which you can ultimately agree. One area you both can almost certainly agree upon is wanting the relationship to be conflict-free, wanting the relationship to be better. This can be the case whether you're a professional or a family member.

If you have been using reflective listening and strategic empathy, your loved one is going to feel that you are an *ally* rather than an *adversary* and getting answers to such questions will be a lot easier than it may sound. When you put aside *your* agenda for the time being, you can find a great deal of common ground.

For example, if the answer to the question about what happened after the medicine was stopped was, "I had more energy but also I couldn't sleep and got scared," you can agree with that observation without linking it to having a mental illness.

At this point in the process, you will have come to know some possible motivations your loved one has to accept treatment (e.g., "sleep better," "feel less scared," "get a job," "stay out of the hospital," "stop my family from bothering me"). These may be reasons that have nothing to do with the belief he or she has a mental illness. You will know what his short- and long-term goals are because you will have talked about them together. And, with this knowledge, you will now be able to present the idea that treatment might help him to achieve *his* goals. I can't emphasize this enough—*your suggestions should have nothing to do with the notion that your loved one has a mental illness.*

Relationships that are respectful and non-judgmental lead to acceptance of treatment.

Finally, whenever you find areas of agreement and you talk about them together, you're strengthening the relationship. Research shows that when you talk about things you agree on, you're usually speaking in a respectful and non-judgmental way. And when you have a relationship with someone that is marked by mutual respect and lack of judgment, it turns out that's one of the best predictors of who will accept treatment and stay with it long-term. In other words, relationships that are respectful and non-judgmental lead to acceptance of treatment.

Partner

Forming a partnership to achieve *shared* goals is one of the most satisfying tools you will use. Once you know the areas where you can agree (e.g., staying out of the hospital, getting a job, reducing tension and conflict with your family), you can now collaborate on accomplishing those goals. Unlike the previous techniques, this one involves both of you making an explicit decision to work together, to become teammates striving for the same goal. *You* may call the prize "recovery from illness," while your loved one calls it "getting a job," but the names are irrelevant to arriving at a shared plan of action that will, more often than not, include accepting treatment and services.

6

Listen

In my LEAP seminars, I always ask, "Why would anyone want to listen to you if he felt you had not first listened to him? Quid pro quo."

This important psychological principle—which is the cornerstone of the LEAP method for breaking an impasse—is far from new. More than 2,000 years ago, the Roman poet Publilius Syrus said, "We are interested in others when they are interested in us." Psychologists who are expert in conflict resolution and marriage and family therapy have written about this fundamental principle for decades. Dale Carnegie, author of the 80-year-old best-seller *How to Win Friends and Influence People*, writes, "Philosophers have been speculating on the rules of human relations for thousands of years, and out of all that speculation, there has evolved only one important precept. It is not new. It is as old as history. Zoroaster taught it to his followers in Persia twenty-five hundred years ago. Confucius preached it in China twenty-four centuries ago. Jesus taught it among the stony hills of Judea nineteen centuries ago. Jesus summed it up in one thought—probably the most important rule in human relations: "Do unto others as you would have others do unto you."

More recently, the authors of *Getting to Yes, The 7 Habits of Highly Effective People, Good to Great, How to Argue and Win Every Time* and other insightful observers of human relations have all emphasized this same fundamental principle of persuasion and cooperation. But despite the ancient lineage and popular dissemination of this simple and logical truth, it is too often overlooked when we are lured into an "I'm right, you're wrong" situation and end up thrashing around like fish caught on the end of a line, certain that if we try just hard enough (i.e., speak more loudly or repeat our position once again), we will win. And sometimes we *do* succeed in bending the other person to our will, but not without doing some damage. Listening with genuine curiosity and respect is the key to not getting stuck in this trap and making it possible for the other person to care about your opinion.

It was 7:30 a.m., and morning rounds had begun on the ward where I worked as an attending psychologist. The entire day shift was seated in a circle around the room. Doctors, nurses, social workers and assorted students were, or soon would be, repeating this ritual on inpatient psychiatric wards all over the country, indeed, all over the world.

The chief of the unit, a psychiatrist, called the meeting to order and then Marie, the head nurse, took over. She began by reviewing how each patient had fared the night before. When she came to Samantha, a 40-year-old single woman with chronic schizophrenia, she paused and sighed before beginning. "Samantha Green, stable on six milligrams of Risperdal and detoxed. She slept well last night and is ready for discharge today. Jo Anna," she asked the senior social worker, "do you want to fill everyone in on the discharge plan?"

"Sure. It's a real gem," responded Jo Anna sarcastically. "Samantha is going back to her parents' house and has an outpatient appointment with her doctor set for a week from today. She's been given a list of AA (Alcoholics Anonymous) meetings near her. Mr. and Mrs. Greene are picking her up at noon and she's walking out the door with a one-week supply of medication."

"You don't sound too pleased with the plan," I said.

"It's nothing personal," she replied, knowing that Samantha and her parents also had an appointment with me for a family meeting. "The plan is all right—it's Samantha I'm not pleased with!" She paused. "Look, we all know what's going to happen. Call me cynical, but I'll bet you ten dollars she stops taking her medication before the end of the month and she'll be back here before you know it. She needs long-term hospitalization, not another trip through the revolving door."

Samantha had been admitted to the hospital four times in the past year. Each episode of illness had been triggered when she secretly stopped taking her medication. Her parents would notice her talking to herself and start to worry that she was not taking her pills. Her mother would then ask if this was so, and Samantha would invariably deny it, even though she had not taken the pills for weeks. By the time the truth came out, it was usually too late and she needed to be hospitalized.

To my ears, Jo Anna's lack of faith in Samantha, her parents, and in me was neither cynical nor insulting. Given Jo Anna's experience and perspective, she would have been foolish to expect anything more than she did. However, if Jo Anna had known what I knew, she might have shared my optimism for Samantha and her family.

I knew why Samantha didn't want to take psychiatric drugs. It had taken some effort to uncover the true reasons, but with that knowledge and a good idea of what Samantha wanted out of life, I knew I could help her stay on the medication, in treatment, and out of the hospital. But Jo Anna and the rest of the hospital staff hadn't learned what I had, because they were focusing on other things.

In the best case scenarios families are also involved in the hospital's discharge plan, but patients with anosognosia all too often forbid contact with family.

In today's climate of managed care and increasing advances in drug therapies for serious mental illness and addictions, mental health professionals working in hospitals have become increasingly specialized. Psychiatrists evaluate health and symptoms and order medications. Psychologists working on inpatient wards typically perform psychological assessments and, less often, do therapy. Nurses dispense medications, monitor patients' health and safety, and provide education about illnesses and treatments offered. Social workers evaluate the patients' discharge needs and make arrangements for outpatient treatment and, if needed, residence. In the best case scenarios, families are also involved in the hospital's discharge plan, but patients with anosognosia all too often forbid contact with family members.

As a psychologist working with persons who have serious mental illness and addictions, I know a good deal about the interventions and medications used to treat these disorders, but I don't prescribe drugs. My job is different. Understanding the person and how the illness has affected his sense of self and goals is one of my areas of focus. And that is why I was optimistic about stopping the revolving door Samantha was stuck inside.

Unlike the others, I knew how Samantha experienced being ill and what she thought about the drugs and sobriety we were "pushing" on her. I also had a clear understanding of what it was she wanted out of life, and that knowledge had helped me to get her to agree to a trial of the medication as an outpatient and to attend thirty consecutive days of AA meetings (I had suggested three times that number but she wouldn't agree so I didn't push it). Unlike the other times she'd been hospitalized, Samantha was not agreeing to these meetings and to taking the medicine to placate us so she could get out. She was agreeing to continue (for a time) to see if it could help her achieve one of her goals. In other words, I had been doing a lot of listening, and what I had learned gave me a foothold with Samantha and reason to have hope.

Building a Treatment Agreement

The cornerstone of building a treatment agreement that will work and outlast your direct involvement is cut from the quarry of your loved one's sense of who she is, what she believes she is capable of doing, and what she wants out of life. Unless you know its shape, color, texture, and strength, you will be unable to build on this foundation. Each stone you lay will topple and fall to the ground unless you have listened and learned about *her* experience. Specifically, focusing on what's relevant, you want to ask about her:

- beliefs about having a mental illness
- beliefs about having an addiction
- experience and attitudes about treatment
- concept of what she can and cannot do
- hopes and expectations for the future

In the next three chapters, I will show you how to put your knowledge of these areas to practical use. But before we get there, you have to know your loved one's answers to each of these questions. And, because serious mental illness and/or addiction often changes the way people communicate with one another and what each person wants to talk about, there are some common pitfalls you'll need to avoid. The best way to do that is by learning how to use *reflective listening*.

LEAP® Reflective Listening

We all know how to listen. But I'm not talking about "everyday listening." I'm talking about a very specific form of pure *reflective* listening (i.e., LEAP® Reflective Listening), which is very different.

|||||||||||||||||||||||||||||||||||||||||||||||||||||||||||||||||||||||||||||||||||||||||||||||||||||||||||||||||||||||||||||||||||||||||||||||||||||||||||||||||||||

When you're doing it right, you're asking a lot of questions.
You sound like a journalist conducting an interview.

|||||||||||||||||||||||||||||||||||||||||||||||||||||||||||||||||||||||||||||||||||||||||||||||||||||||||||||||||||||||||||||||||||||||||||||||||||||||||||||||||||||

Reflective listening has, as its sole purpose, understanding what the other person is trying to convey and then communicating that understanding back to that other person without commenting or reacting in any way. It is an active, rather than passive process — your role is purely that of a listener who wants to get it right. When you're doing it right, you're asking a lot of questions. You sound like a journalist conducting an interview.

I'll give you an example of how and why something that seems so simple doesn't come naturally. All my life, people have told me I am a naturally good listener. As a psychotherapist, I pride myself on my ability to listen and understand other people's experiences. But everything I thought I knew about listening was put to the test the first few times I tried to converse with people who had anosognosia about serious mental illness and/or addiction.

I was 23 years old when I took a job as a psychiatric technician (a.k.a. nursing aide) on an inpatient psychiatric ward at the University of Arizona Medical Center. My brother Henry's first psychotic episode had occurred less than a year before, and despite his rambling speech and crazy ideas, I could still understand him. My experience with my brother had given me a lot of confidence. *I have listened to many bizarre things,* I thought. *I can do this.*

As a psychiatric technician, I was responsible for assessing, among other things, how agitated, depressed, manic, suicidal, substance abusing, or dangerous my patients were. I was also charged with determining whether my patients were following the prescribed treatment plan. Every conversation had a hidden agenda.

My very first admission evaluation was with Barbara, a 42-year-old woman who was in the throes of a grandiose delusion and irritable manic episode. She was talking a mile a minute about her power to read minds, her supernatural abilities, the alien implant in her brain that had given her these powers, and the fact that she didn't need to be in the hospital. And she was very angry about being there.

With a bright red hospital-issued clipboard on my knee, I diligently started with the list of questions that were printed neatly in rows on the evaluation form. "Can you tell me why you came to the hospital?"

"Can you tell me why *you* came to the hospital?" She mimicked me with disdain, effectively humiliating me for being a rookie.

I tried to recover my composure. "I am sorry. You were brought here by your husband. That's right, isn't it?"

"I am sorry. You were brought here by your husband. That's right, isn't it?" she echoed sarcastically.

Stating the obvious, I said, "It sounds like you don't want to talk right now. I am sorry, but I have to get through these questions." I pleaded with her, despite the fact that I was feeling even more humiliated and was also starting to get angry.

"I don't give a shit about your f__king questions!"

"I'm sorry, but I really do need to get through these questions."

"Grow up, little boy. You better realize who you're dealing with here. You don't know what you've gotten yourself into and you are in way over your head. Way over your head. Maybe I'll *have* your head. I could, you know. It's as easy as snapping my fingers or blinking an eye or squashing the wings of a butterfly!" She shouted at me in rapid fire before bursting into hysterical laughter.

My agenda was moot, my face a bright shade of red. I know, because she made a point of telling me as I was excusing myself and trying to walk—not run—out the door. I was scared and angry. I went to the nurses' station and plopped down next to Nancy, the charge nurse.

"You got that done fast," she said.

"Not really. I didn't get much done at all."

"She wouldn't answer your questions?"

"No. All she did was mimic my every word and threaten me."

"Threaten you?!"

"Not exactly. At least not in reality. She was threatening me with her supernatural delusional powers."

"Well, it seems like she may not be able to answer these questions right now. What did you learn about her from just sitting in the room?"

"Well, she's angry and doesn't want to be here. She's in denial. She's manic, irritable, and grandiose. And she doesn't want to talk to me. Maybe someone else should give it a shot."

"No. She's your patient. I just gave her some medicine—give her a couple of hours to calm down a little, then try again. Only this time, don't bring in the admission form. Start by asking her if there's anything she would like to say. Let her talk about why she thinks she shouldn't be here and see where it goes. Ask her questions about that. That seems to be where she's at, Xavier. Look for an opening to tell her you're sorry she's here."

"God knows *I'm* sorry she's here!" I said, joking and feeling better. I saw the wisdom in Nancy's advice. I followed her suggestions and ultimately learned quite a bit about Barbara. But it took putting my questions and agenda on the back burner for me to listen to what she was feeling about being forced to be a "mental patient" in a psychiatric hospital. As a result, I was able to get my form filled out. Some questions were not answered, but the essentials were covered. (I will tell you more about Barbara

later. But for now, I want to focus on the other elements of LEAP®
Reflective Listening.)

*To do it right, you have to drop your agenda. Your only goals are
to understand what your loved one is saying and
to convey that understanding.*

It's hard to listen reflectively in the face of all the distracting
"noise" of psychosis or the insane rationalizations of addiction,
especially if you are pursuing an agenda and trying to follow a
timetable. To do it right, you have to drop your agenda as I did
with Barbara. *Your* only goals are to understand what your loved
one is saying and to convey that understanding.

This is very hard to do at first, but it's not impossible and
actually gets quite easy once you "unlearn" your natural bad habits.
Reflective listening is a skill and, as with any skill, once you know
the basic principles, all you need to do is practice to get it right. To
start, here are seven guidelines for LEAP® Reflective Listening:

Seven Guidelines for LEAP® Reflective Listening

1. *Make it Safe*
2. *Know Your Fears*
3. *Stop Pushing Your Agenda*
4. *Let it Be and Don't Judge*
5. *Respect What You've Heard*
6. *Find Workable Problems*
7. *Write the Headlines*

1. Make it Safe

During the first few years he was ill, my brother Henry never
wanted to talk to me about the medicine he was prescribed. He
didn't *feel safe*. As you will learn later on, we argued a lot for

many years, going round and round on the issues of whether he was sick and needed to take medicine. We got into what I call the *denial dance,* which creates pessimistic expectations about talking.

Let me tell you about one of my first experiences with this.

> *My brother had just come home from the hospital and was doing well. The medication obviously helped him, but within a day of his getting home, I found it in the garbage can. Naturally, I asked him why he'd thrown it out.*
>
> *"I'm okay now," he explained. "I don't need it anymore."*
>
> *This ran counter to everything he was told in the hospital, so I made a point of reminding him. "But the doctor said you're probably going to have to be on this medicine for the rest of your life. You can't stop taking it!"*
>
> *"He didn't say that."*
>
> *"Sure he did! I was at the family meeting, remember?"*
>
> *"No, he said I had to take it while I was in the hospital."*
>
> *"Then why did he give you a bottle of pills to take home?" I argued, trying to prove him wrong.*
>
> *"That's just in case I get sick again. I'm fine now."*
>
> *"No, that's not what he said."*
>
> *"Yes, it is."*
>
> *"Henry, why are you being so stubborn? You know I'm right!" I said.*
>
> *"It's my business. Leave me alone."*
>
> *"When you got sick it became everyone's business. And besides, I'm worried."*
>
> *"You don't have to worry about me. I'm fine."*
>
> *"You're fine now, but you won't be if you don't stay on the medicine."*
>
> *"That's not what the doctor said!"*
>
> *"Then let's call him and I'll prove it!"*
>
> *"I don't want to talk about it! Just leave me alone," he said as he walked away.*

With every dose of "reality" I tried to give him, Henry countered with more argument and denials. And with every go-round, we both became angrier and angrier. I thought he was being stubborn, irresponsible and immature. My accusations and threat to prove him wrong made him even angrier and more defensive. My natural instinct to confront what I thought was denial was completely ineffective and only made things worse. We got caught in a cycle of confrontation and denial that pushed us further apart and, not surprisingly, left my brother feeling that it was not safe to talk with me about these issues. The end result of conversations like this was that he walked away. (The dance *always* ends in avoidance.)

Henry said it best after one of our early arguments. "Why should I talk to you about this? You don't care about what I think. You're just going to tell me I'm wrong and need to see a shrink!"

It wasn't until I was in training to become a psychologist that I finally understood that my brother wasn't simply being stubborn or irresponsible. Armed with more knowledge and experience, I reflected on how I had talked to him and realized I had played a big role in getting him to stop talking and start sneaking (e.g., when he secretly threw his medicine in the garbage while claiming he was still taking it).

I made him feel unsafe. He knew that if he said he wasn't sick and didn't need medication, I was going to argue with him. And he was right! Sometimes I did it gently, but as the years wore on and he became what mental health workers call a "frequent flyer" or "revolving door patient," I was often harsh in my confrontation of what I thought was simple denial (I didn't yet know about anosognosia). Once, I even planned an intervention involving several family members and Henry's social worker. We all, gently but powerfully told him he was in denial. One by one, we told him he had schizophrenia and needed to take psychiatric drugs to get better.

Now imagine if that happened to you (assuming you do not have schizophrenia, which was exactly Henry's point of view). Imagine that this conversation followed on the heels of dozens more like it. Would you really be interested in explaining, once again, that there was nothing wrong with you and you didn't need treatment? No. Better to walk away or, if you can't, shut up and pretend to agree in order to get the conversation over with quickly.

> *"I am sorry for not listening to you. I understand why you don't want to talk about this anymore."*

So how do we make it safe to talk? First, set aside a special time. It can be over a cup of coffee, a walk, on top of a Ferris wheel! Anywhere. What matters is how you introduce the conversation.

If you've had arguments in the past, you need to apologize and acknowledge that you made your loved one feel unsafe. You can say something like, "I am sorry for not listening to you. I understand why you don't want to talk about this anymore." And then normalize his reaction to you by saying something like, "If I were in your shoes, I would feel the same way." When you apologize for jumping in with your opinion (which I call *reactive* listening) and admit you would feel the same way he does, you make it safe to talk.

But there's more. You have to promise *not to do it again* and make good on that promise. "I want to hear more about why you hate the medicine and I promise I won't do anything but listen and try to get a better understanding of your view on this. I promise not to give my opinion."

You might be thinking, "Wait a minute! How can you help someone in denial if you are not going to tell him the truth? Don't you have to help him see the problem and the solution?"

Yes...and no. How long have you tried to convince your loved one that he's mentally ill or has an addiction? Remember Einstein's definition of insanity? Have you been trying for six months? One year? Two years? Longer than two years? And have you succeeded? I'm assuming you haven't and that's why you're reading this book. So, perhaps it's time to try a different approach.

Advice can be perceived as either welcome or unwelcome, respectful or disrespectful, loving or patronizing.

Advice is a funny thing. It can be perceived as either welcome or unwelcome, respectful or disrespectful, loving or patronizing. What determines how the advice will be received?

Here's an example. Women who are pregnant often complain about how complete strangers walk up to them and give them unsolicited advice. Sometimes it's humorous; usually it's irritating. But almost always, they ignore the free advice because it was uninvited, patronizing, and felt intrusive.

And yet, *every* woman I have talked to about this experience admits that she had at least one friend or relative whose counsel she sought and listened to. *That's* the difference between *solicited* and *unsolicited* advice. Advice that someone *has asked for* carries far more weight than advice we give without being asked. So, when you promise to *not* give your advice because your main goal is to listen and learn, you gain instant credibility. And I guarantee, as strange as this may sound, that you will be asked for your opinion, and most likely, far sooner than you would like.

So, apologize for not listening well enough, promise you will listen without comment, and *keep the promise*. To succeed, you will need to discover why you have been afraid to listen in this way, because if you don't, the same fears that kept you from reflective listening in the past will trip you up going forward.

2. Know Your Fears

Whenever I teach LEAP® Reflective Listening to a new group of people I am reminded how much more similar than different we all are. On the outside, all sorts of differences jump out at me—the man in the business suit sitting near the one in the "Guns Don't Kill People, People Kill People!" T-shirt; the large loud woman; and the meek, diminutive one.

People of all shapes, sizes, religions, races, and politics come to LEAP seminars because they all have a deep desire to help a loved one who has anosognosia (is in "denial"). They also have the same fear about taking that first step, the fear that, "I will make it worse if I listen the way Dr. Amador says I should."

During these seminars, I define reflective listening just as I did above. Then I ask for a volunteer. I did this role-play with Gwen in Halifax, Canada. Her job, as I explained it to her, was simply to listen to me as I role-played a delusional patient...and then reflect what she had heard.

> Gwen looked confident as I began the role-play. Speaking fast and sounding very angry and scared, I said, "I am not sick, there's nothing wrong with me. I'm not taking that medicine because it will kill me. It's poison. If you want to help me, then help me with the people upstairs."
>
> "What about the people upstairs?" she asked, without reflecting what I had just said.
>
> "Every night at eight o'clock, they walk across the floor of their apartment to the bathroom. I hear them flush the toilet and I know what they're doing! They're communicating with the people who have been trying to kill me!"
>
> Gwen, who had been nodding as I explained the problem, answered, "So it sounds like the people upstairs are disturbing you. They're making a lot of noise?"
>
> Seeing that she was done, I asked the audience, "Did Gwen reflect back what my patient said?" Immediately, numerous hands

shot up. One after the other, they described how she had not. They saw what Gwen could not see in the moment – although she had responded in the form of a question, as I had recommended, she had not reflected a single thing I had said. The closest she came was mentioning that I was "disturbed" by the people upstairs. In fact, however, I wasn't disturbed. I was scared and angry and it had nothing to do with their being "noisy" neighbors. The noise didn't bother me – it was their use of the toilet as a signal device to communicate with people who were trying to kill me!

The audience was able to see that she had not reflected what I had said, but few did better themselves when they tried their hand at it. Like Gwen, they omitted mentioning the "crazy" facts. The closest anyone came was acknowledging that the toilet flushing was a signal to the people in the building who wanted to "kill me." But they all avoided talking about my anosognosia, my belief that the medicine was poison, and the stranger, more paranoid delusion that there was a conspiracy of fellow tenants who were planning my murder.

After reassuring my volunteers that I used to make the same mistakes with my brother before I learned LEAP Reflective Listening, I modeled the correct way to do it. Playing the role of the listener now, I said, "So, Xavier, tell me if I got this right. You're not sick and don't need to take medicine. It's poison. If I could help you with anything it would be with your neighbors. Every night they're communicating with the people in your building that are trying to kill you. Do I have that right?"

Not even halfway through saying this, I could see several people squirming in their seats, shaking their heads, and frowning. I said, "I know that many of you are very uncomfortable with what I just said. What makes you so uneasy?"

One man practically shouted.

"You're reinforcing the denial!"

"You can't tell this guy his medicine is poison. He'll never take it!" Gwen added.

"What else worries you?" I asked the group.

"You worsened the delusion; now you're going to get drawn into it. He's going to want you to do something about his neighbors," another man offered.

A woman I knew to be a social worker raised her hand. "This goes against everything I was taught. You can't collude with a delusion like that. You'll reinforce it!"

I turned to the group. "Was anyone feeling okay about what I did?"

An elderly woman in the front row raised her hand. "I thought it was fine," she said. "He's going to want to talk with you because you are talking about what's important *to him*. He doesn't believe he's crazy and thinks people are trying to kill him, for gosh sake!"

"So why do you think the rest of them are so uncomfortable with my reflecting all that back to him?" I asked.

She slowly turned around to look at the audience, then, turning to face me again, she said simply, "They're chicken," and sat back down. After the laughter subsided, I thanked my unexpected accomplice and elaborated on her wise observation.

When you're facing someone who rigidly holds irrational beliefs, you gain nothing by disagreeing.

First, I never agreed with his beliefs about being sick, the medicine, or the paranoid ideas. By prefacing and ending my statements with questions ("Did I get this right?" or "Do I have that right?"), I was free to use my patient's own words. In no way did I challenge his beliefs. Why should I? He's delusional!

Rather, I showed him through my actions that I wanted only to listen to him and understand. I have never talked anyone out of a delusion, and, to my knowledge, I have never talked anyone *into* one either. The point is, when you're facing someone who rigidly holds irrational beliefs, you gain nothing by disagreeing. More importantly, you lose that person's willingness to talk about the problem.

There *are*, however, a few pitfalls you have to watch out for. One is when the person asks, "So it sounds like you agree with me. Do you?" Or the flip side of the same coin: "Why are you acting like you believe me?"

Actually, these questions offer an important opportunity, which I'll talk about in the following chapter. For now, I ask that you trust me—and for the time being, focus on uncovering what *your* fears are.

3. Stop Pushing Your Agenda.

I know your agenda is to help someone you're worried about. And you have specific ideas about how the help should come. But because the person has anosognosia, they're already expecting unwelcome advice for a problem they don't believe they have. You need to keep *your* agenda to yourself!

When reflectively listening, the only stated agenda you should have is your desire to listen, understand and learn. When a person trusts that you will not pontificate about what he should and should not be doing, he will be more apt to agree to talk about certain "hot" topics (e.g., his refusal to seek professional help).

Agreeing on an agenda is easy if you follow the lead of the person who has anosognosia. This is how I was finally able to engage Barbara. What she wanted to talk about was how furious she was for being forced into the hospital when she wasn't mentally ill. If the person you're trying to talk to is upset about having to take medicine, ask him about his *feelings*, not about the medicine or your belief that he should take it. You can say, "I'd like to understand why you hate taking the medicine. Would you mind talking with me about that? I promise I won't pressure you or bug you—I really just want to understand how you feel about it."

Try it once with any hot topic and see what happens.

4. Let it Be.

If the discussion turns into an argument and you feel the denial dance coming on, stop! If your loved one becomes accusatory, saying something like, "You don't care about me, all you're thinking about is yourself," just let it be. Don't fan the flames by disagreeing and defending yourself.

Sometimes mental illness creates "thought disorder," making it especially difficult for others to follow the person's train of thought. It's annoying and frustrating. When talking with someone who has thought disorder or disorganized speech, be careful that you don't inadvertently impose order on the chaos, because usually you will get it wrong.

In other words, let it be and focus on listening *differently* instead of on trying to impose order. Listen for the feelings behind the words and reflect back the emotion. When you understand the underlying emotions, you will discover what the person truly cares about most and what motivates him.

What is especially important is not to judge what you've heard. Judgments can be subtle—from a raised eyebrow to vocal inflection.

When dealing with addiction, it's hard to listen to the denials and irrational justifications of "bad behavior" stemming from substance abuse. But in the case of mental illness and addiction, if you want to make progress you need to put aside your judgments and save them for when your loved one is ready and able to hear your point of view.

5. Respect what you've heard.

When you make it a point to communicate your understanding of what you've just heard without reacting to it, you convey your respect for the other person's point of view. By not defending or disagreeing, you create an environment that's inherently respectful. You also deflate anger. When you echo what you've heard without comment or criticism, you stop that "I'm right, you're wrong!" cycle dead in its tracks. Think of it this way: Would you really be interested in hearing the opinion of someone you've been arguing with if you felt he or she hadn't listened to *your* views?

6. Find Workable Problems.

Everyone in denial or with anosognosia knows he has at least one big problem and that problem is *you* – you and everyone else who is telling him he needs help!

He will have other problems you can uncover as well. Understanding how the person who has anosognosia sees himself and his beliefs about what's not working in his life is the key to unlocking the isolation and building a relationship with someone who recognizes he is in trouble, has problems, and maybe could use your help. The help he needs can only be found through such a relationship *if he is unaware of the illness.*

Consequently, you first need to learn what *he* thinks the problem is. Now, I'm not talking about mental illness or addiction. I am talking about the problems *he defines.* How does *he* describe the problems? What does *he* say he needs to fix them? Without understanding what he thinks is wrong and what he thinks needs to change, you will be powerless.

For example, my brother never agreed that he had schizophrenia, but he *did* think that being forced into a psychiatric hospital again and again was a big problem. I couldn't have agreed with him more. Once you find a problem you can work on together (e.g., Henry and I agreed that avoiding another hospitalization was a very good thing), you have common ground and with that comes a new relationship—one in which your opinion starts to matter. It is also vital that you find out what he wants out of life—in the short term and long term—without being judgmental. So, if he says, "I just need everyone off my back and a job!" it wouldn't be a good idea to say something like "You're putting the cart before the horse because you need treatment first." That's exactly what I used to say to my brother—communicating that he needed to take medicine before he started thinking about a job.

In summary, *don't be judgmental*. You need to find out what is important to your loved one and let him know that you've heard and value his opinion.

Finally, the last guideline is to do what I call "writing down the headlines."

7. Write Down the Headlines.

I started out by telling you that to do this right, you need to approach your loved one the way a journalist would. That means not only asking questions without injecting your criticism or other opinions, but also discovering a theme and figuring out what the "headlines" are.

So, after a conversation in which you've been reflectively listening, think of the front page of a newspaper and literally write down the headlines. If you can, write them down in front of the person (I will give you examples of how to do this later) so that you know you are both on the same page about what's important to him.

What are "headlines"? Headlines are the problems the person believes he has (not the problems *you* say he has) and the things that motivate him to change (those that are most important to *him*). Ultimately, you are going to work together on the problem as *he* defines it and link it to the help *you* believe he needs. And you will do this by harnessing what motivates *him*.

To illustrate these listening guidelines, I offer the following two examples from families I have worked with. The first is an example of how *not* to listen while the second provides an excellent lesson on how to do it right. And by "right," I simply mean using LEAP Reflective Listening — not conveying judgment or defensiveness — and instead communicating respect for what you just heard. Both examples are drawn from my work supervising therapists in training on an inpatient psychiatric ward. Because my students typically bring video tapes of their sessions with families to our supervision meetings, I can comment on both the therapist's and the family members' listening skills.

Ineffective Listening

It was 3 o'clock and Dr. Brian Greene, a second-year resident in psychiatry, was meeting with Matt Blackburn and his parents. Matt is the 26-year-old man I first told you about in Chapter 1, who lives at home with his parents. As you may recall, he was admitted to the hospital believing he was a close confidant of the U.S. president. He also believed that God had chosen him as His special messenger to world leaders, that the CIA was trying to assassinate him, and that his mother was trying to sabotage his mission (this last belief was not entirely delusional).

When he was admitted to the hospital, he was also hearing voices and had thought disorder (rambling, disconnected thoughts strung together so that when he spoke it was often difficult to make sense of what he was saying). After two weeks of treatment at Columbia University, his speech was more cogent and the voices had quieted down a bit, thanks to the medication he had received. He still had the same delusional beliefs, but the drugs helped relieve the pressure he felt to act on them (e.g., go to Washington to meet with the president).

The meeting was called by Dr. Greene to discuss what Matt would do after being discharged from the hospital. "Mr. Blackburn, Mrs. Blackburn," Brian said to each as he shook their hands, "Please come in and have a seat." Matt was already seated at the end of a long table in the patient dining room.

His mother circled the table to reach her son and bent down to give him a kiss. Mr. Blackburn immediately sat down in the nearest chair, which was also the farthest from Matt, and started asking questions of Dr. Greene. "I know we're supposed to be talking about Matt's discharge, but don't you think he needs to stay here longer? I don't think he's ready to come home yet."

"There's really nothing more we can offer him here, Mr. Blackburn," Brian answered. (In truth, it probably would have helped Matt to stay another week, but his insurance had run out.)

"Well, I don't think he's ready and neither does his mother!"

"Hold on," Mrs. Blackburn said, "I didn't say that exactly. Of course, we want you to come home," she said, directing her last comment to Matt. "We're just worried about what's going to happen next."

Seizing the opportunity, Brian began. "Matt has an appointment later this week with a doctor in our outpatient clinic. He has enough medicine with him to last until that appointment and the hospital's day program has accepted him. He can start there as soon as the doctor has seen him."

"This is exactly what I was afraid of," said Matt's father to his wife. Then he turned to face Brian and added, "I don't want to be negative, Dr. Greene, but he'll never go to that appointment and he won't go to this day program you're talking about. He doesn't think there's anything wrong with him. We need a better plan than this. Matt won't take his pills and he doesn't like hanging around the people in these programs. He says they're all crazy!"

Brian rightly turned to Matt. "What do you have to say about all this?"

Matt responded loudly, while looking down at the table. "I said I'd go. I'll go!"

"That's what you promised us before, Matt," said his father in a kinder tone. "But when we get home, you disappear into your room and you don't go anywhere."

"It's different this time. I'll go! I just want to get out of here and get a job and my own place."

"Are you sure you'll go?" his mother asked, looking worried.

"Yeah, Mom, don't worry. I'll go. I really will. Okay?"

Matt's father didn't look convinced, but his mother and doctor looked, if not convinced, at least relieved by what they had just heard.

Let's review the seven listening guidelines I gave above.

1. Did They Make It Safe?

Brian and Matt's family did set aside a special time to talk but did not make the conversation "special" in the way I described above. There was no acknowledgment of their differing views and no apology for previous attempts to convince Matt he was in denial and mentally ill. No one explained that he or she wanted only to hear Matt's views on the discharge plan. And no promise was made to refrain from giving unsolicited advice.

Instead, the old argument was immediately raised by his father and the battle lines drawn. The result was that Matt got defensive and then did what you and I would have done had we, like Matt, been through this a hundred times before. He lied and said he would go to the appointment. He lied to get his parents and his doctor off his back and to get released from the hospital.

2. Did They Know Their Fears?

On the surface, Matt's father and mother both appeared to be in touch with the fear they felt going into this conversation. But they were not. They were aware of their fear that their son would continue his career as a "frequent flyer" or revolving-door patient—but they had no awareness of the specific fear they had about this conversation, which was that they would make things worse if they didn't make their views known once again.

Although she did it more gently than her husband, Matt's mother also laid down the battle lines. She wanted her son to stay in the hospital longer. She made it very clear she thought he was still very sick. Both parents and Dr. Greene, for that matter, felt compelled by their fears to once again tell Matt, *as if hearing it once again would make a dent in his denial,* that he was ill and needed professional help. And yet, all three knew that Matt was not going to follow up with the clinic appointment.

They could have talked about that with him directly. But to do that they would have had to make it safe for him to talk and not let fear rule the conversation.

3. Did They Stop Pushing Their Agenda?

Matt was about to leave yet another hospitalization, and his parents and doctor knew he would not follow through with their recommendations because he never had before. But that didn't stop the three of them from pushing their hopeless agenda anyway.

Dr. Greene wanted to communicate the details of the post-hospital treatment plans and "seal the deal" so to speak (even though he admitted to me later that he knew Matt would never follow through with the plan as it had been presented to him).

Matt wanted to leave the hospital and was willing, if that's what it took, to take medicine for the time being. How long he was willing to stay on the medicine was never determined because Matt did not trust his doctor or parents enough to be forthcoming and reveal what his true feelings were.

Mr. Blackburn openly predicted that his son would stay on the medicine for less than one week while Brian naïvely hoped that Matt would be willing to follow doctor's orders for months to come. Mr. Blackburn was pursuing an agenda, which was trying to convince Brian to hold Matt in the hospital longer. And although Mrs. Blackburn was focused on the same agenda, she was preoccupied with her guilt and with not wanting to hurt or anger Matt.

What was Matt's agenda? No one asked, so we really don't know, although I found out later.

4. Did They Let It Be?

Matt was not offering his opinion or saying he would not take his pills. At least, not directly. So, there was little in the meeting for his doctor and parents to react to. But his parents were reacting to things Matt had said and done in the past. His father was angry from the start, not only because the hospital was discharging his son, whom he felt was too ill to come home, but also because he didn't believe Matt was telling the truth. When Matt said he'd go to his appointment and take his medicine, his father reacted essentially by calling him a liar. ("That's what you promised us before, but when we get home you disappear into your room and you don't go anywhere.") Although more subtle, Matt's mother also reacted to his reassurances with disbelief.

5. Did They Respect What They'd Heard?

No one reflected, or echoed, back to Matt what they understood him to be saying. Matt's views on whether he was ill and needed treatment were not respected. There was at least one missed opportunity. When Matt said, "This time is different," his doctor or parents could have replied, "So, Matt, I want to understand. You're saying this time is different. Is that right?"

If such a question had been asked, not with anger or skepticism but with genuine curiosity, Matt would have answered yes, his defenses would have dropped a notch, and he would have told them something very important. This time really *was* different for him. He truly did not want to come back to the hospital ever again, certainly not the way he had this time (his parents had called the police, who brought him to the hospital against his will and in handcuffs).

And if they had echoed back what they heard and Matt had felt they truly understood, a problem they all shared could have been identified. They could have worked together *to keep him out of the hospital.*

From Matt's perspective, his parents were the reason for his hospitalization and the handcuffs. From theirs, it was the mental illness and Matt's stubbornness. But they all agreed that no one wanted him to end up in the hospital again (even the insurance company would have agreed to that). If they had taken the opportunity to show respect, Matt might have dropped his defenses and the volume on everyone's anger would have been reduced.

Let me give you a feel for what I am talking about. Brian was Matt's doctor and I was Brian's supervisor, so sometimes I met with the two of them together. During one of these meetings, Matt described the terror he'd felt when the police brought him to the hospital. He had never felt so scared before and he never wanted to feel that way again. And he had grown tired of being hospitalized again and again. I asked him why he thought his parents had called the police and he answered, "Because they think I'm sick."

"But Matt, that doesn't tell me *why* they would put you through this."

"They think I'm sick and need to be in the looney bin, that's why."

"Let me ask the question differently. What's motivating them to do this to you? Do they hate you?"

"No."

"Do they want to hurt you?"

"I don't know. I don't think so."

"Then why would they call the police on their son?"

"They're afraid, I guess."

"Matt, let me see if I have this right. Your parents called the police to bring you to the hospital against your will, not because they hate you or want to hurt you, but because they're afraid. Do I have that right?"

"Yeah. That's it."

"What are they afraid about?"

"They're afraid I'll get hurt."

"Now, I know you disagree with them on this, but before we talk about that, let me see if I am following you so far. Your parents were afraid you would get hurt so they wanted you in the hospital to keep you safe. Is that right?" He nodded. "What does that tell you about how your mom and dad feel about you?"

"They love me."

"So, you have a big problem here, don't you? How do you convince your parents to stop calling the police and throwing you in the hospital? I mean, you can't convince them to stop loving you, can you?"

"No," he said, smiling.

"Then what?"

"I can't convince them there's nothing wrong with me. You guys have them all brainwashed!" We both laughed at his reminder that people like me — doctors — were at the root of his problem.

"No. And they can't convince you that you're sick. So there you are. What could you work on together?"

"I guess reassuring them so they don't get scared and call the police."

"How can you do that?"

"There's nothing I could do to convince them."

"Nothing?"

"Well, no...not nothing. I guess I could take the medicine."

"But if I understand you, you're not sick. Why would you take medicine if there's nothing wrong with you?"

"To keep them off my back!" he said, sounding a little defeated.

This conversation, though valuable, would have been priceless had Matt had it with his parents. But because they were afraid and unable to echo what they heard, they missed a chance to find common ground with their son and work on the problem they all agreed *Matt* had (i.e., hospitalizations against his will were bad). By redefining the problem so that it was no longer about the question of whether or not he was sick and needed help and clarifying that he knew his "misguided" parents were motivated by love, Matt could have translated the impossible problem he had into one that was workable.

6. Did They Find Workable Problems?

When it came to defining the problem, Matt, his parents, and Dr. Greene were talking apples and oranges. Matt saw the problem as his parents, the police who listened to them, and the shrinks who had convinced his mother and father he was ill.

Matt's parents and Dr. Greene saw the problem as his being stubborn, immature, and defensive—he was not taking any responsibility for the illness he *clearly* had.

On the other hand, Matt and I had easily found at least one workable problem. We agreed that the only problem anyone would be willing to work on with him was how to keep him out of the hospital. Identifying a problem we could work on together opened up a way for us to work together as allies rather than adversaries.

After his parents left, I briefly met with Matt and Dr. Greene and said: "Well, you know it's your choice, Matt. You know what I think, and I can't force you to do something you don't believe in. I wouldn't want to do that even if I could, unless, of course, you were in danger, which you're not in right now. I respect your right to make this decision for yourself.

"I know you told Dr. Greene and your parents that you would stay on the medicine. But if you change your mind—and if I had to guess I'd guess you will since you don't believe you're sick—I hope you will pay close attention to what happens next. It's your life. Don't just have an opinion about the medication—prove to yourself whether your opinion is right or wrong."

"I already said I'd take the pills!" he responded defensively, probably because I was implying that I didn't believe the reassurances he'd given Dr. Greene and his parents.

"Okay, I will take you at your word. But I have to say something. If it were me, I wouldn't take the medicine." Seeing that Brian looked mortified by what I had just said, I turned to him. "Dr. Greene, do you have something to say? You look like you might have a different view on this."

"Well, I don't think you really meant that if you were in Matt's shoes, you wouldn't take the medicine."

"That's exactly what I meant."

Brian frowned and seemed to be searching for words when Matt saved him by asking me, "So, you don't think I need the drugs?"

"I promise I will answer your question, but can I tell you later?" Matt nodded, letting me delay.

"What I said is that if I were *you*, I wouldn't take them after I leave the hospital. I've been listening to you and your views on this and it's obvious that *your* truth is that you don't have a mental illness and you feel strongly you shouldn't be taking medicine for an illness you don't have.

"That sounds like common sense to me. Who would take pills if they didn't think they needed them? What would be the point? If I believed those things, I wouldn't be planning on taking the medicine. If I were in your shoes, I would say whatever it took to get out of here and then follow my own compass. Isn't that really where you are? You can tell me and you will still go home today. It won't change a thing."

"I would *never* do that," Matt said facetiously, a smile spreading across his face. I smiled back as we both recognized and shared the truth of what he would do once the door closed behind him.

"Hypothetically then, if you *do* stop taking the medicine, ask yourself these three questions: What stays the same? What gets worse? What gets better?"

"Yeah. The pluses and minuses."

"Exactly. So, you know what I'm talking about?"

"Yeah. It's my life. I hold the key and it's up to me to decide."

"Right. Now, you've decided you really don't want to take the medicine. You don't need it— right?"

"Yeah," he admitted sheepishly. "But I will anyway. Everyone wants me to, so I will."

"Well, I don't know if everyone wants you to, but you know my opinion. I hope that you will. But if you decide to stop, I want you to know I respect that this is your life and your right."

"Yeah, but you'll think I'm stupid."

"No, I won't. But I might think you made a bad decision for yourself given your goal of staying away from the police and out of the hospital."

"You're the doctor. You would know."

"It's true I am a doctor, but the fact is your opinion is far more important than mine. You're the one that's going to decide. Anything else you want to add?" He looked surprised. "No I guess not."

"Well, good luck." I stood up, extended my hand, and added, "I hope I never see you again."

"Same here," Matt replied. We both laughed as we shook hands. We both knew that if I saw Matt, it would be because he was back in the hospital. Keeping him out of the hospital and in his life was something we both wholeheartedly agreed upon.

7. Did They Write the Headlines?

No one appeared to pay any attention to the headlines, much less write them down. Of course, writing down what Matt had to say would have been awkward in this situation because his doctor and parents had never practiced the LEAP technique with him. It's true that Brian often took notes during their sessions, but they were almost entirely about symptoms he was observing. They were not going to be shared with Matt as they were really only for Brian's eyes. He rarely recorded Matt's subjective experience of the problem (his parents, the police, and the "shrinks") or recorded statements that revealed what was important to him, what motivated him (staying out of the hospital, getting a job and a place of his own). But it would have been easy to ask, "Is it all right with you if I write down what you're talking about? I think it's important."

Effective Listening

Dr. Ivan Kohut, a third-year resident in psychiatry, was meeting with Vicky, the 45-year-old woman with bipolar disorder you heard about in Chapter 2. Her husband Scott was also present. Vicky had spent the last two weeks in the hospital following a manic episode during which she had taken her two children on a three-day "road trip" to Mount Desert Island, Acadia National Park, in Maine.

The first night of the trip was especially disturbing because Scott had no idea where his family had gone—until Vicky called him at 11:00 p.m. to explain that she wanted their children to experience the same spiritual awakening she was having. God, she told him, had instructed her to take them to the top of Cadillac Mountain because it was the highest point on the East coast, and had told her that once they were there, he would come to them.

Having gone through two previous manic episodes with Vicky over the course of their marriage, Scott figured out what was happening much more quickly than he had in the past. During the phone call, he begged her to come home, but she refused. When he told her he thought she was becoming sick again, she abruptly hung up the phone. Scott immediately called the police in the area she had phoned from, but they told him there wasn't much they could do except to "keep an eye out for her car." They suggested he call the National Park Headquarters in Maine.

With the help of Vicky's psychiatrist, Scott was able to convince the park rangers to intercept his wife when she arrived. He then flew up to Maine and after much cajoling and threats of involuntary commitment, he got her agreement to return to New York and go to the hospital.

From both Scott's and Vicky's perspective, the drive back was nightmarish. The children—as children often do—were unconsciously running interference by misbehaving. Their fights and tantrums, together with Vicky's rapid-fire speech and grandiose proclamations, made for an excruciatingly long drive home.

After greeting the couple, Ivan sat down and began. "What would the two of you like to talk about today? I have two things I'd like to put on our agenda. How about you, Vicky?"

"When do I get out of here? That's the only thing I'd like to talk about," she said.

"Okay. Scott, how about you?"

"Well, I have the same question. And I also want to talk about her medications."

"Anything else? Either of you?"

"No," Vicky answered quickly.

Scott thought a minute. "I suppose not. Maybe more will occur to me as we talk."

"Good, then. My two agenda items are similar," said Ivan. "I want to report on how I think Vicky is doing and then ask her how she feels about the discharge plan. So, that's basically three items: One, when does Vicky get out of here; two, my view on how she's doing; and three, Vicky's opinion of the plan we put together for after she leaves. If it's okay with the two of you, I'd like to get the second item out of the way first."

Vicky and Scott both nodded their approval.

Addressing Vicky, Ivan said, "I think you are doing much better than when we first met two weeks ago. Back then you were sleeping about two to four hours a night, your thoughts were racing, your speech was pressured, you were euphoric, extremely irritable, and you had some unusual thoughts about God and supernatural abilities you felt he had given you. Right now your sleep is back to normal, your thoughts aren't racing, and your speech isn't pressured. You don't need me to describe your mood. How would *you* describe your mood over the last week?"

"Kind of constricted. I'm not as happy and I don't get irritated so easily. I'm not depressed."

"Do you miss the happy feeling?"

"You know I do, Dr. Kohut! Wouldn't you?"

"Absolutely." Noting the smile on her face, he added, "But it looks to me like you can still feel happy. It's the *extreme* happiness, the high, that's gone. Yes?"

"That's true," she answered.

"So, in a nutshell, I think you're ready to go home the day after tomorrow."

Vicky looked surprised. "Why didn't you tell me that this morning when we met?"

"I suppose you don't remember, but I told you I had to discuss it with the team first. I wanted everyone's input. We generally make these decisions by consensus, and the consensus is that you're much improved and can go home. Scott, any opinion about this?"

"Not really. I expected it. I see that she's getting back to normal. But I guess I'm not clear on what happens next. What can we do to keep this from happening again?"

"Good segue to the last item on our agenda — what happens next with respect to your treatment." Ivan addressed Vicky once again. "I'd like to see you in the clinic once a week for the next couple of months, and then maybe drop down to once a month. I don't want to change anything about the medication you're taking right now. I'd like to see how you do over the next couple of weeks, then re-evaluate and discuss if we should make any adjustments. What are your thoughts about what should happen next?"

Vicky laughed. "Does it really matter? Everyone thinks I should stay on medication."

"Of course, it matters!" Scott replied, a little irritated and defensive.

"You're the boss here, even if it doesn't seem that way now," Ivan added.

"What are you talking about?" asked Vicky.

"I am talking about the fact that what your husband and I think you should do doesn't amount to a hill of beans compared to what *you* think you should do. If you believe that the medications have done their job and want to stop taking them, you will. I can't stop you and neither can your husband."

"Then why am I here? I don't *feel* like the boss."

"That's because you lost a lot of control when the disorder you have flared up. It caused you to do things that worried a lot of people and motivated them to take control away from you. But now you've got the illness under control again and you're back in the driver's seat."

"If that's true, then I don't want to take these drugs for more than a month or two."

Using LEAP reflective listening, Ivan said, "So, if I understand you, you don't want to take these drugs for more than two months at the most. Right?"

"Yes."

Scott interrupted. "Wait a minute! That's how she got into this mess in the first place. Every doctor she's seen, including you, has told us she will very likely have to stay on these medications for the rest of her life."

"If she doesn't want to have another flare-up, yes, that's true. That is my opinion. Also, the medications will help to keep her from becoming depressed again. I'm not contradicting myself. I'm saying something else. It's Vicky's choice, not yours or mine. But the choices you make," he added, looking at Vicky, "will have consequences."

"You make it sound so ominous," she replied.

"I think the consequences of stopping your treatment will be very negative. You know what my professional recommendation is and what your last psychiatrist felt. You know what your husband and your family would like. But what you believe is what you will ultimately do. And I *have* to respect that. But I am curious about one thing. Why don't you think you will need the medications? Just this morning you told me they've been very helpful over the past few weeks. Were you just 'yessing' me or did you really mean it?"

"I meant it. They've done their job. But I'm better now."

"So, you see yourself as cured of bipolar disorder?"

"Well, I'm not sure I have bipolar disorder. But whatever was going on, yes, the medications helped calm me down. So, yes, the problem is solved. Why would I want to be on these drugs for the rest of my life when the problem doesn't exist anymore?"

"So, what you're saying," Ivan began, "is that you had some kind of problem—not bipolar disorder—that the drugs helped you with. And now that the problem is solved, you don't want to keep taking the medication. Right?"

"Right."

"Want my opinion on what you just said?"

"I already know it."

"Actually, it may surprise you."

"Shoot."

"What you propose is certainly possible," Ivan said to the couples' surprise. "How about we make a deal. If you decide six months from now that you still want to go off your medications, we can give it a try. But I won't have any part of it if we're not meeting regularly."

"Why would you do that? You already told me you think I have to stay on these medications forever."

"Because your opinion is the only one that ultimately determines whether or not you stay in treatment. I am willing to work with you to prove what you believe even though I don't share the same belief."

Vicky agreed to meet with Dr. Kohut regularly. And although Scott looked worried, he agreed with the plan as well.

1. Did They Make It Safe?

Did Ivan make it safe for Vicky to talk? Yes. He made it clear that he wanted to hear Vicky's views on the treatment and was actually reluctant to tell her his views, which she already knew. She understood she could talk about her belief that she was not sick and didn't need treatment without her doctor contradicting her. She also knew that Ivan would keep her husband from jumping down her throat. Ivan made it clear that her opinion was the only one that really mattered at the moment. It was more important than his and Scott's opinion.

2. Did They Know Their Fears?

Scott got nervous and went on the attack for a moment when Ivan acknowledged, without argument, Vicky's desire to stop taking the medicine. Otherwise, Scott did a great job of listening passively as his wife and doctor discussed her views on the problem and what she needed. In previous meetings, Ivan had worked with Scott to help him recognize where he was powerless and would benefit from acceptance. Where he was powerless was in convincing his wife she had bipolar disorder and needed to be on medication for the rest of her life. He hadn't succeeded in four years, and Ivan helped him to recognize what was obvious — he wasn't going to suddenly succeed now by continuing the argument. Where he had power was in repairing their relationship so that she would feel he was once again her ally, on her team, and that they were working on the same problems together.

Ivan was clear about his fears and understood that he had nothing to lose by listening and not contradicting Vicky's views. He knew he would not harm her by allowing her to be honest, by not contradicting her views without her permission (he always asked her if he could give his opinion before he gave it), and he had nothing to lose and a lot to gain by actively listening.

3. Did They Stop Pushing Their Agenda?

Not only did they agree on an agenda but over the course of their conversation, Ivan repeatedly checked back with Vicky and her husband to ensure that there wasn't anything else either of them wanted to talk about. The main agenda was understanding Vicky's views and working with how she experienced all this.

4. Did They Let it Be?

Ivan did not react emotionally to Vicky's statement that she wanted to stop taking medication. Neither did Scott, except during the one brief moment when his fears caught him off guard. Neither Ivan nor Scott jumped in with their opinions to refute Vicky's statements that she was no longer ill, no longer needed medicine, and planned to stop taking it. They let her opinions stand. They respected her point of view. When Ivan *did* offer his opinion, he empowered Vicky by first asking if it was okay with her for him to tell her what he thought.

5. Did They Respect What They Heard?

Ivan did this repeatedly, often rephrasing things Vicky had said to ensure that he "got it right." He prefaced his reflective statements by indicating that he just wanted to be sure he understood her correctly ("Let me see if I got this right?"), used her words without comment or criticism, and then asked her if he'd understood correctly. He acknowledged that he understood and *genuinely* respected her point of view.

6. Did They Find Workable Problems?

Vicky felt that the medications were a short-term treatment, like antibiotics for an infection, rather than a long-term treatment, like insulin for diabetes. The good news is that Vicky had some awareness, though nowhere near as much as her family and doctor would have liked. She understood that the drugs helped her when she had symptoms but didn't understand that the medicine could prevent the symptoms from returning when she was feeling well.

Although Ivan understood that statistically it was highly unlikely she could stop without getting sick again, there was a small chance that she could. He also understood that until the day Vicky "owned" the treatment, until she found a reason that made sense to *her* to stay in treatment, she never would. Her problem, which he was willing to help her with for the time being, was taking the medicine. But he would work with her on this only if she stayed in therapy with him, allowed Scott to come to some of the sessions, and took some responsibility for paying attention to what happened when she stopped taking the medicine.

By agreeing to work with her on the problem as *she* defined it, he kept her in therapy and on the medication for a longer period of time than if he had insisted the treatment was "a life sentence," as she had once described it. He also laid the foundation for her discovering reasons to continue in treatment. It's important to note that the foundation I am referring to did not require Vicky to be *aware* she has an illness that requires life-long treatment.

7. Did They Write the Headlines?

Ivan not only wrote down what they had agreed to do about the medications but asked permission to do so before starting. This was important because it emphasized Ivan's wish to *collaborate rather than pontificate*. By asking, he also underscored that Vicky would be in charge after she left the hospital. He wasn't afraid to acknowledge his own powerlessness.

By doing that, he reminded Vicky that the choice to continue treatment was hers, as was the responsibility for the consequences that would follow her decision. The "headlines" were that she wanted off the medications and that she understood they helped her when her thoughts were racing, when she wasn't sleeping, and when she got tired out (these were the things she saw as problems even though she didn't think she still had an illness).

In summary, LEAP reflective listening is an active process. It involves asking many questions and not reacting to what you are hearing. You should think of yourself as a scientist trying to unravel a mystery. Your task is to gain a clear idea of what your loved one's experience of the illness and treatment and of what your help is. Once you know how he experiences the idea of having a mental illness and taking psychiatric drugs, you will have acquired vital knowledge you need in order to build an agreement about treatment.

The "Danger" of Listening Reflectively

Very likely, the person you are listening to reflectively and without judgment will make the mistake of thinking you believe what he believes (about not being sick, not needing medications, not having a substance abuse problem, or even about the CIA conspiracy he has a delusion about). Or, he may believe you are willing to talk to his family about not being sick and needing any form of treatment. I touch on this problem at various points in this book. It's the reason most people are afraid of reflective listening—they think it's somehow dangerous.

Delay, Opinion and Apology Tools

To help with this concern I will introduce you to three new tools that are not in the "LEAP" acronym (but are among the seven LEAP tools): The *Delay*, *Opinion* and *Apology* tools. These tools will allow you to use reflective listening without falling prey to the difficult interactions, or traps, described above. If you like using acronyms like I do to remember things, you may have noticed these three letters spell out DOA. That sounds terrible! In fact, I believe our relationships with people who have anosognosia for their condition is often dead on arrival (DOA) when we don't use these techniques. So I like DOA. I will talk about these three techniques again later but let me lay them out for you here concisely.

Delay Tool

You want to delay giving your *contrary* opinion whenever possible (about delusions, desire to not accept treatment, etc.) for as long as possible to preserve the alliance you are building, delay the hurt your answer will cause, and perhaps most importantly, shift the *locus of control* to the person who is asking for your opinion (i.e., from passively hearing an opinion to actively asking for it).

So in terms of learning to use LEAP, the longer you are able to delay giving your contrary opinions, the more the person you're helping will experience you as respecting his opinion and therefore more obligated he will feel to respect yours. At the very least, he will be more likely to hear you out without getting immediately defensive. If he has to solicit your opinion, the more in control he will feel and less defensive he will be when he hears it. The harder he has to work to hear your opinion, the more highly he will value it, even if he still disagrees. For these reasons, your opinion will have more weight.

When you delay, try the following: first *honor the question* by promising to answer it, *attempt to change the topic* to something else that's important to the person, and *ask permission* to do so. Here are some examples that include all three elements (the promise, the diversion to a meaningful topic, and the request for permission to change the topic):

- *I promise I'll tell you whether I think you are sick. But first, if it's OK with you, I would like to hear more about how you ended up in the hospital, that seems really important to you. Would that be all right if I tell you later?*

- *I will answer your question about the CIA. Can I ask you to give me some more details about what happened first? Would that be OK?*

- *You've asked me many times whether I think you're delusional. I promise to answer, but if it's OK with you, before I tell you what I see, could you tell me more about what happened when your parents called the police? Would that be OK?*

- *I promise to tell you whether I think you're really an alcoholic. Before I do would you be willing to tell me more about your attempts to control your drinking? Can we do that?*

- *I promise to answer your question about whether you should stop taking medicine. Before I do, I want you to know that I believe your opinion about this is far more important than mine. Can you tell me more about that and I will tell you my opinion after?*

When I use this communication tool—in my experience— the person I am attempting to help often forgets their original question and the conversation continues without my having to give a show-stopping contrary opinion!

I recall once when I delayed saying, "Your opinion about treatment is far more important than mine," and my patient said to me, "But you're the doctor! Your opinion has got to be more important!"

I disagreed and told him so. "When we're done talking and you walk out this door, you are in the driver's seat. Your opinion is what will determine what you do and where you go, and the choices you make. Your opinion is far more important than mine."

By saying this, I was empowering him—More accurately, I was recognizing and emphasizing his real power of self-determination—while humbling myself. More important, it was coming from my heart. I believed it. As you can imagine, this made me and my opinion a lot less threatening to him than I, or it, would have been otherwise. And when I did give my opinion about treatment, using the LEAP tool I describe next, it was met without any defensiveness or anger. On the contrary, he thanked me for being honest with him.

Opinion Tool: The Three "A's" for Giving Your Opinion

Sometimes, even after you've listened and empathized, the other person won't ask you what you think. This is rare in my experience. If it happens to you, consider two possibilities. One is that you have not used the tools you've learned as effectively as you could...and the other is that the person likes talking so much that he simply isn't interested in what you have to say. If it's the latter, you can ask if he or she would be willing to hear your perspective. You can say something like, "After listening to you, I have a much better picture of your views on this. Can I tell you what *I* think?"

I've never heard of anyone who has used the listening and empathy tools receiving a "no" in answer to this question, and I don't believe you will either. But whether you have been asked for your opinion repeatedly and delayed giving it, or you have had to offer it because the person doesn't ask (despite being cooled down and feeling listened to and respected) the *way* you deliver your opinion will determine whether it throws more fuel on the fire or continues to douse the flames.

If you want to get past the impasse, there is a new tool you now need to add to your tool belt. I often use all three elements of this tool together, but sometimes you need only one or two to get the job done. I call these my "A" tools — it makes them easier to remember and they are powerful tools you can use whenever you're arguing or negotiating. I like to think of these tools as *soft*, like felt or a goose-down pillow. Sometimes I think of them as airbags. In other words, they are tools that help to soften the blow and save lives...or, at least, relationships.

The "three A's" to use when giving your contrary opinions are *apologize* (for your opinion's emotional impact), *acknowledge* (that you could be wrong), and *agree* (to disagree).

Apologize

Apologizing may be the last thing you think you need or want to do at this point. After all, the other person has been asking you (hopefully more than once) what you think. You're only doing what she's asked. In fact, you may think that if you need to apologize for anything it would be for having delayed so long — but that's not the way it works.

Keep in mind the reason you delayed in the first place: because you're aware that when you *do* give your opinion, it could damage the trust you've so carefully been building. When you finally admit that you don't agree, the other person is likely to be disappointed, to feel somehow betrayed, and to get angry all over again. So what you need to indicate is that you understand all this and *apologize*, because you do truly wish what you believe didn't make her feel that way.

I'm *not* suggesting you apologize for the opinion you're about to offer (e.g., "Yes I think you may have bipolar disorder...") but for the feelings it might engender. You're not saying you're sorry you feel this way, but rather that you're sorry that what you have to say may make him or her feel upset. What you should say is something like, "Before I tell you what I think about this, I want to apologize because what I think might feel hurtful or disappointing."

Understanding that difference ought to make the process easier for you. If you still feel unable to apologize, you're probably still too angry, and you need to take a few deep breaths, step back—if only for a moment—and think about why you're doing this in the first place. In my view, you're never going to win on the strength of your arguments or opinions. *You're going to win on the strength of your relationship.* And that's why you're giving your opinion in this way—to minimize harm to, if not to strengthen, the relationship.

When you *do* apologize, just be sure that you *don't* use the word "but," as in, "I apologize if this is going to upset you, *but* I think..." I mentioned this before but want to emphasize it here again because it is so important. When you use the word *but*, it's like hitting the mute button on the other person's ears. People who are in a disagreement (including you) typically stop listening when they hear the word "but." Not only are they incapable of hearing you—the most likely outcome is that you'll just revert to "butting" heads all over again.

Acknowledge

What is it that you need to acknowledge? Certainly not that you still think you're right (although, ultimately, that's more or less what you're going to be saying). Rather, you need to acknowledge that you're not infallible and you might be wrong — even though you clearly don't think so. (And you're *not* going to say *that!*) So, after you apologize, say something like, "Also, I could be wrong about this. I don't know everything." For example, "I want to start by apologizing because my opinion about the medicine might be hurtful and *I could be wrong.*" That's what the first two A tools can sound like together.

When you acknowledge your fallibility, you are, first of all, indicating that you are flexible. If you can be flexible, you're more likely to trigger some flexibility in the other person. If you're rigid and dogmatic, you're equally likely to trigger that. Remember that LEAP is all about *giving* in order to *receive*.

Acknowledging that you could possibly be wrong is also a way to convey respect because you are not insisting that you are wise and the other person is ignorant. It's the same principle Benjamin Franklin wrote about in his autobiography:

"I made it a rule to forbear all direct contradiction to the sentiment of others, and all positive assertion of my own. I even forbade myself the use of every word or expression in the language that imported a fix'd opinion...for these fifty years past no one has ever heard a dogmatical expression escape me."

If it worked for Benjamin Franklin, who broke many seemingly insurmountable impasses, it can work for you.

Agree

I've already said that you're not going to be agreeing with the other person's opinion. So what is this about?

Here, you're going to ask her to agree to disagree. In other words, you'll be indicating that you respect her opinion and hope that she'll respect yours. "I hope we can just agree to disagree on this. I respect your point of view and I won't try to talk you out of it. I hope you can respect mine."

Another way to agree to disagree is to say, "I hope we don't have to argue about this because there's so much we agree on I'd rather focus on that." Another example is to say, "I don't need to be right. I just want to have a good relationship with you."

Using the "three A's" (Apologize, Acknowledge and Agree) is far easier than it might appear at first glance. When my brother Henry asked me if I thought he had schizophrenia, I said: "I'm sorry because this might hurt your feelings. I want you to know I could be wrong. I don't know everything, but yes, I think you might have something like schizophrenia. I hope we don't have to argue about this Henry — I respect your opinion and I hope you can respect mine. Can we agree to just disagree?"

Did you see any or all of the "three A's"?

Here is a shorter example. I was working with someone with bipolar disorder who asked me several times, "Do you think I should take the medicine?" After delaying repeatedly, I finally answered, "I'm sorry I feel this way and I could be wrong, I just hope we can agree to disagree. I think you ought to try it for a little while longer." Do you see how I used all three A's? If not, go back and read my answer again. Furthermore, I didn't insist on educating my patient about bipolar disorder and the need to take medicine for the rest of his life.

Apology Tool

Although an apology is in the last tool (the three A's for giving your opinion), apologies can and should be used in other instances. The goal of apologizing is to convey genuine humility and respect. The ultimate goal is to further your goal of creating a relationship that leads to the acceptance of treatment and other suggestions you have made. What kind of things might you take the opportunity to apologize for? Here are some examples.

You might apologize for:

- Not sharing the same belief about…
- Disappointing the person
- Annoying the person with "too much" reflective listening
- Not doing what was asked of you
- An involuntary treatment you supported/initiated
- Boundaries and/or restrictions you have put in place

What else might you want to apologize for? Give this some thought with an eye toward communicating compassion, empathy and respect rather than turning yourself into a doormat!

In summary, the main point of the DOA tools is to be genuinely humble, help the person save face, and preserve the relationship you've been building. Remember, you will win on the strength of your *relationship* rather than on the strength of your argument.

7

Empathize

A few years after he first became ill, my brother and I were talking about one of his medications, Haldol. He hated Haldol (a.k.a. haloperidol). As I listened to his complaints, I understood for the first time some of the frustration he felt about taking these medications. I recall saying something along the lines of, "I can see why you don't like these drugs. They make you feel stiff and groggy." The conversation stands out in my mind because for the first time, we were calmly talking *about the medication* and listening to one another instead of arguing.

Usually our conversations on this topic were a disaster. I would hold my ground and pontificate about why he should take the medications prescribed for him and about how immature it was of him not to accept the fact that he was ill. Brothers can often be that way, but after working for a year as a therapy aide on an inpatient psychiatric ward, I was beginning to learn how important it was to really listen.

As I listened, I couldn't help beginning to empathize. I loved Henry, and when someone you love is in pain, it's hard not to empathize. Learning to listen led to empathy. And my empathy ultimately resulted in my brother showing a real interest in *my thoughts* about the illness and the medications he was sure he did not need.

The LEAP empathy tool is not everyday empathy. As shall be seen, it is *strategic* empathy focused on those feelings the person has that most of us fail to acknowledge—much less empathize with.

These are among the most important feelings to connect with because they are the feelings that drive people with mental illness away from their loved ones and therapists.

When *you* feel empathy and convey it, your loved one will likely feel understood and respected. When *you* convey that you understand how your loved one is feeling, his or her defensiveness will decrease and openness to your opinion will increase. If *you* have listened reflectively to your loved one's experience of his illness and the prescribed treatment, you will naturally begin to empathize.

Communicating empathy can be tricky when you're talking to someone who has a psychotic illness, however. Many people worry that they should not empathize with certain feelings, such as anger about being forced to take medicine, fear of treatment, feeling victimized because they are certain they are not ill (have anosognosia), or feelings connected to delusions when, in fact, these are among the most important feelings to connect with—because they are the feelings that drive people with mental illness away from their loved ones and therapists.

Strategic Empathy

You must first learn what it is you should be empathizing with. The short answer is "any *feeling* your loved one is willing to reveal." But there are certain feelings that are particularly important for you to empathize with. Whether they are rational ("I am so tired of everybody telling me I am sick!") or irrational ("The C.I.A. has implanted microchips in the capsules so they can track me! I'm scared!"), you want to be sure to empathize with feelings stemming from anosognosia, delusions and desires. For example:

> **Frustrations** (about pressure from family and healthcare workers to accept being mentally ill or addicted, accept treatment, and about unrealistic personal goals that have not been met).
>
> **Fears** (about treatment, being stigmatized, and failing).
>
> **Distress** (attributed to medications, such as gaining weight or feeling groggy, slowed down, less creative, etc.).
>
> **Desires** (to work, get married, have children, return to school, stay out of the hospital, etc.).

A magical thing happens when you combine reflective listening with strategic empathy. Your loved one will ask you what you think! I can almost guarantee this will happen.

For example, remember the conversation I had with Matt and his doctor? Matt, whom everyone knew didn't think he was mentally ill, had just insincerely promised to take his medicine when he left the hospital. And I said, "Okay. I will take you at your word. But I have to say that if it were me, I wouldn't take the medicine." He opened up to me then and was more honest about not wanting to take the drugs. When he did that, I focused on empathizing with his feelings about taking them. I said, "You sound angry that everyone is pushing these drugs on you. Are you?" He agreed, then eventually asked me, "So, you don't think I need the drugs?"

You saw my answer to that question, but what you didn't know was that the time was ripe for me to give him my opinion (using the three A's). He was about to leave the hospital, and it was my last chance to talk with him. Most of the time, however, when someone asks my opinion about a delusion, about whether I think he's mentally ill or needs medications, I try to delay answering.

For example, one patient was convinced that his mother was poisoning his food. I listened and empathized, and he then asked me if I believed it was actually happening. Our conversation about this began with my saying, "So, if I understand you correctly, your mother has been poisoning your food. Do I have that right?"

"Yes!"

"How do you feel about that?"

"Are you serious? How would *you* feel?"

"I would feel—and I think anyone would feel—scared and angry," I replied.

"So, do you believe it? Are you going to do something about it?" he asked.

I didn't answer his questions at that point, although I did later. I delayed answering as long as I could. The take home point is: *Listen and empathize and you will be asked your opinion and it will matter.* Remember, an opinion that has been asked for carries far more weight than one that is forced on a person who is arguing with you.

Dolores

Dolores, who has had schizophrenia for nearly 20 years, told me that she didn't need medication or a day treatment program because there was nothing wrong with her. What did Dolores feel she needed? More than anything else, she wanted a job. She was frustrated that she did not have a job—and also with her family, who told her she couldn't work. Her family was being reasonably pessimistic. The fact is that Dolores had been unable to keep a job for more than a few days at a time and she had been employed only a handful of times over the past twenty years.

By the time I met her, Dolores, like many individuals with serious mental illness who don't know they're ill, had been hospitalized many times—in her case, two to four times per year. Although she almost always signed herself into the hospital voluntarily, she would do this only after receiving tremendous pressure from her family. When I talked with her about what she planned to do when she left the hospital this time, she told me simply, "Get a job."

If you were her therapist and discussing her plans, you might be tempted (as I was early in my career) to focus on the irrationality of the idea. After all, she had a long history of poor adherence to her medication and multiple hospitalizations — there was no reason to believe that her longstanding pattern of unemployment was about to change. You might understandably think that talking about her reluctance to stay in treatment would be more beneficial than encouraging or agreeing with her irrational plan to get a job.

The problem was that Dolores had absolutely no interest in talking about drugs, day treatment programs, or doctors' appointments. Would you want to talk about those things if you were certain that you were not ill?

So, instead of going that route, I began our talk about her plans for the future by empathizing with what she was feeling at that moment. "You want to get a job when you leave?"

"I'm going to work on Wall Street," she answered.

"Why Wall Street?" I asked, ignoring how far-fetched her plan was.

"I want to make a lot of money. I need to have my own money."

I reflected her statement back to her. "If I understood you, it's important to you to have your own money and you can do that by working on Wall Street. Is that right?"

"Yes, I hate having to ask my parent's for money."

"How come?"

"It makes me feel like a child. My little sister [who was in her 30's at the time] is a stockbroker and you should see her house. I'm the big sister. I should be making money too!"

I checked to see if I understood her feelings and, at the same time, communicated my empathy. "It sounds like asking for money makes you feel embarrassed or even a little humiliated. Am I right about that?"

"It does. Wouldn't you be embarrassed?" she asked.

"Yes, I think I would feel that way." Sensing an opening, I added, "Can I ask you something?"

"What?"

Careful not to add to her humiliation and raise her defenses, I asked, "Why do you think you haven't worked very much?" (Note that I *didn't* ask, "Why is it you've only worked about twelve days in your entire adult life?")

"Because I'm always in the damn hospital!"

"Is being in the hospital keeping you from work?"

"I'm angry about being in the hospital so much. I want to get on with my life and I can't if I'm in a damn hospital."

"So, it's much more than frustration you feel. It makes you angry. Yes?" I asked, nodding my head.

"Very angry," she answered, more calmly this time.

I pushed ahead. "How do you feel about the fact that it's been hard to find work?"

"Sometimes I want to scream!"

"That sounds infuriating. Is it?"

"No. It's frustrating," she said, correcting my misperception.

"So, it's frustrating. Sorry I got that wrong."

"That's okay."

During this brief exchange, I empathized with Dolores's feelings of *humiliation*, her deep *desire* to work, and her *frustration* with being unable to work. Did you notice that nearly everything I said was in the form of a question? That is how you should do LEAP reflective listening and LEAP empathy. Also, by making a statement about my understanding of her feelings and asking if I had it right, I was able to make sure I understood what she meant when she said she wanted to scream. I communicated my empathy for what she was feeling and allowed her to be in control of the conversation.

Also, by asking questions instead of commenting on what she had to say (e.g., "What you're planning isn't realistic..."), I learned what was important to *Dolores*, what was uppermost on *her* mind, and how *she* was feeling. I created a window of opportunity, which I later used to discuss what role, if any, she felt treatment might play in what *she* wanted to accomplish (i.e., staying out of the hospital and working on Wall Street).

Whenever you want to facilitate change in another person, you must first become his friend (i.e., someone he trusts). Whenever you convey empathy for another person's experience, he feels understood, respected, and more trusting. Because you understand the other person's point of view and how he feels about his situation, there is nothing to argue about. What he feels is what he feels—nothing less, nothing more. There's no one to push against. Consequently, he becomes less defensive and more open to hearing your perspective. And, more often than not, he will ask either: "So, do you believe me?" Or, "Why are you acting like you believe me? You don't believe me, do you?"

These questions are opposite sides of the same coin—a coin you want to handle carefully as your answer is vital to where you want to go.

With LEAP strategic empathy you are focusing on those feelings that most people ignore.

Remember that toolbelt I asked you to imagine? Well, you had empathy on the left side of your toolbelt even before you picked this book up. With LEAP empathy on the right side of your toolbelt, we're now talking about focused *strategic empathy*. What do I mean by that? You are now paying special attention to those feelings of a loved one or patient that are stemming from things like delusions, anosognosia, and their deepest desires (whether or not they are realistic). So you empathize with feelings such as *frustration* about family who are telling the person their mentally ill, *fear* of being in treatment, *excitement* about what you see as an unattainable career, etc.

With LEAP strategic empathy, you are focusing on those feelings that most people ignore. And when you do that, you are building a bridge to someone who is often very lonely and alone with their feelings. Once you've built that bridge, you're ready to start looking for areas where you can agree and work together.

8

Agree

One of the questions I'm typically asked when conducting LEAP workshops is, "This sounds great, but who has time to do this?"

At this point, you may be feeling the same way. In fact, it takes no more time to use LEAP than what you have probably been doing all along. Think of all the time you've wasted arguing or attempting to coerce the person you've been trying to help into accepting treatment. In my experience, LEAP doesn't take more time, and the research I cited earlier confirms that impression.

Hopefully, you are now reassured on this count and eager to learn the next tool. Having listened carefully to your loved one's attitudes and feelings about treatment and having conveyed your empathy, you have undoubtedly found areas where the two of you can agree.

I didn't share Matt's beliefs that God had chosen him as his special messenger to the president, that the CIA was trying to assassinate him, or that he was not ill. But we did agree on at least one thing — *that it was important to keep him out of the hospital.* Dolores and I agreed on something similar, and that her goal was to get a job. Although I didn't think it likely that work was right around the corner for her, I *did* believe she could start taking steps in that direction. Vicky and Dr. Kohut agreed to examine together whether she truly needed to take medication after she left the hospital. My brother Henry and I agreed that when he took his medication regularly, he stayed out of the hospital, the voices he heard bothered him less, he became less fearful, and my mother stopped pressuring him and arguing about taking medication.

When you share the same goals, you can work together instead of being at odds.

Whenever you see a window of opportunity to convey your observations and opinions, always begin with something your loved one already acknowledges and believes. The more common ground you can find, the better. When you share the same goals, you can work together instead of being at odds with one another.

Let's look at how to recognize and use a window of opportunity to find common ground.

Recognizing and Using Windows of Opportunity

Dolores believed the main reason she had not been able to find work was because of her frequent hospitalizations. Although this was certainly part of the reason (you can't work and be in the hospital at the same time), it was the end product of what I believed to be more relevant factors. She, however, had no awareness (i.e., anosognosia) into the more salient reasons she had trouble finding and holding onto a job.

According to her family, Dolores lost the few jobs she was able to get because of the symptoms of her illness. For example, she would begin talking to herself while at work, having quiet conversations with the voices she was hearing. Sometimes she would become paranoid and accuse her bosses and co-workers of plotting against her.

Dolores, however, didn't recognize the symptoms of her

illness, much less the role they played in keeping her unemployed. Instead, she felt certain her numerous stays in the hospital were the root cause of her unemployment.

Consequently, when we talked about her desire to work, I avoided the issue of symptoms or the role they played in her being fired (unless she specifically asked my opinion about this issue). Instead, I focused on the part of the explanation we *did* agree upon—*hospitalizations*. We agreed that being in the hospital made it impossible for her to work. This led to our agreeing on something else that helped me to formulate a treatment agreement she could accept.

Before I tell you more about Dolores, I want to tell you about three things I try to do whenever I see a window of opportunity — when defenses have been lowered and your loved one appears receptive to hearing your views:

1. Normalize the experience. "I would feel the same were if I was in your shoes."
2. Discuss only perceived problems/symptoms. Statements such as, "I can't sleep at night because I'm constantly on guard. I am so afraid that they're going to come and hurt me," describe insomnia and paranoia stemming from a delusion. However, the words insomnia and delusion *should not be used* in your discussions).
3. Agree to disagree. Whenever areas of disagreement are brought to the surface — don't argue!

Dolores was angry and frustrated about being hospitalized so often and about how this interfered with her goal of getting a job. I empathized with her frustration and anger when I said, "It sounds like you feel really frustrated and angry about being in the hospital again."

"Very. I need to get out of the hospital and get back to work. I'm going to go crazy if I stay here much longer."

"You're feeling stir crazy?"

"Yes!"

I followed with, "You know something? We're exactly the same that way. I would go absolutely stir-crazy if I were locked up in a hospital and didn't have a job. In fact, I think anyone would feel that way."

With this small bit of self-disclosure, I was helping to *normalize the experience* Dolores was having. I then asked her if there were any other reasons she was not having luck holding down a job.

Some of her ideas made sense. Others were illogical — if not frankly delusional — and scattered in between were little kernels of awareness into how her disorganized behavior may have contributed to her being fired repeatedly.

Noting these instances of insight, I asked if she wanted my thoughts on *her problem* (notice that we are now talking about a problem *she* perceives). She did.

I began by reflecting to her what she had said earlier. Then, I made a statement in the form of a question. "Well, certainly being in the hospital is interfering with your being able to work. I guess that raises the question of what you can do to stay out of the hospital."

"I don't know. Move away from my family?" she answered wryly.

"Is there any pattern that you've noticed?"

"Well, my father is usually the first one to start picking fights with me. He tells me I'm sick and that I need to go to the hospital. He's always on my back about taking my medications."

"Why is that?"

"He thinks I'm psycho."

"That bothers you?"

"Yeah, it bothers me."

"I can see why that bothers you. Psycho is a pretty derogatory label. Does he actually say that? Does he say you're psycho? Or is that how it feels to you?"

"No, he doesn't say that. He thinks I have a chemical imbalance in my brain."

Here I was normalizing her experience by acknowledging that being called a "psycho" would be upsetting, to say the least, to most anyone. It *is* a derogatory term. I was also asking for clarification. "So, if you were taking your medications, do you think he wouldn't be on your back?"

"I know he wouldn't."

"I see. And when the two of you fight about the medication, it often ends up with you going to the hospital? Is that right?"

"Yes!"

"So, would it be fair to say that there are two advantages to taking these medications? The first being that your father would not be on your back and the second that you would be less likely to go to the hospital?"

"Yes, that's true, I suppose."

I asked her to clarify in order to be certain of exactly what it was she was agreeing to. She said, "If I took the pills, my father would leave me alone and I wouldn't have to come here."

I followed quickly. "What are some of the *disadvantages* to taking medications?"

"I am not a psycho, for one. Also, I hate how much weight I gain whenever I'm on them."

"What else? Are there other side effects or other things about the drugs that you see as disadvantages?"

"They're mind-altering and I don't want to get addicted."

"You are worried about getting addicted?"

"Yes. These are powerful mind-altering drugs," she said.

"They're powerful and they do affect the way you think and feel. Should we put that on the list of disadvantages? That the medications are mind-altering and addictive?" I asked.

"Yes," she answered.

"Any other disadvantages to taking the medicines?" (Notice that I was not trying to convince her that the drugs weren't addictive and that I did not say "*your*" medicines because she didn't see them as hers.)

"It's embarrassing. I don't want anyone to know I am on them."

"Can we write this down so we can keep track?" I asked.

"Sure!"

I took out a pad and pen. "Let me see if I heard the disadvantages correctly. They make you gain weight, feel like a psycho, they're addictive and they're embarrassing. Is that right?"

"Yes, that's right," she said.

"What about the advantages? What I heard was there might be two advantages. Your father would be off your back about taking these medications and you would be in the hospital less often, if at all. Is that right?"

"Yes, you've got it right," she said.

If you're using LEAP, you are always being honest.

I read the list out loud to make sure I reflected everything back to her and asked her to keep thinking about advantages and disadvantages, the costs and benefits of taking the medicine.

You're likely wondering why I didn't correct Dolores's misconception about the medications being addictive. In fact, the ones she was prescribed are not. The reason is that I wanted to avoid conflict and, instead, focus on the areas where we *agreed*. By writing "addictive" down in the "negative" column, I wasn't lying or being dishonest, just recording her perceptions. *If you're using LEAP, you are always being honest.*

It's true she might have come away from our conversation with the erroneous idea that I agreed the medications were addictive because I didn't contradict her or attempt to educate.

But by focusing on what *she* believed the disadvantages of taking the medication were, I was communicating respect, building trust, and aligning myself as an ally rather than as someone who was going to tell her, yet again, that she was wrong.

Dolores visibly relaxed as I spoke. "So you don't think I should take the medication after I leave?"

"Well, no, I didn't say that. You never really asked me for my opinion."

"So...what *is* your opinion, Dr. Amador?"

I welcomed her question because I felt the time was right to tell her what I thought. She wasn't defensive, so I didn't feel the need to delay giving my opinion. "Well, if we're talking about your getting a job, I see the same two advantages that you see. Your father would stop pressuring you and you would stay out of the hospital. So those might be two good reasons to take them. I also see reasons not to take them like gaining weight and the other things we talked about that are on this list."

"So, what's your opinion?"

"I will tell you if you want but it might be disappointing, and I could be wrong. And I am really sorry I feel this way. I wish I didn't feel this way because I don't want to argue with you, but I think you ought to give the medications a try." (Did you see how I used the "three A's" to give my opinion?) I paused for a second. "But I think you should give them a try for the reasons we discussed — *not* because you're psycho. If you take them, you can always change your mind later."

"Why should I try them?"

"Because, at least in my mind, the advantages outweigh the disadvantages. Do you disagree?"

She paused. "I'm not sure."

"Well, let me ask you this. Did I at least answer your question about what my opinion is?"

"Yes. You think I should take them if I want my father off my back and want to stay out of the hospital."

"That's basically right, except *you're* the one who said it would cool things down with your dad and keep you out of the hospital. Not me."

Did you notice that when I gave my opinion and in the conversation that followed, I never once said she should take the medication because she needed it or because she had a mental illness? Instead, I stood firmly on our common ground — all those areas where we *did* agree.

Dolores accepted treatment and in fact, accepted a long-acting injectable medication, not just pills. In Chapter 11, "Medications," I tell you more about why this was preferable to pills. In the meantime, I strongly encourage you to go back and reread our discussion to see if you can identify when I used each LEAP tool.

9

Partner

"How did the psychologist find his wife who was lost in the woods?
He followed the psycho path."

— Henry Amador —
October 1997

Henry and I agreed that being hospitalized was something to be avoided. We also agreed on his goal of getting a job and obtaining more "pocket money" so he could buy soft drinks, cigarettes, or a hamburger if he felt like it.

Although I felt he was much farther away from holding down a job than he did, this difference of opinion was rarely mentioned. Instead, I focused on what we agreed on and avoided those areas where we disagreed (e.g., his having a mental illness).

Sometimes he would try to corner me by saying, "You don't think I can work right now, do you?"

Usually, I was successful in delaying my opinion by saying things like, "I'll tell you what I think if you insist, but what I think doesn't matter. Your opinion is far more important than mine. Can I tell you what I think later?"

Most times, that was enough to move him from his original question to one that would be more fruitful, such as what it would take for him to reach his goal.

In reality, since the onset of his illness, Henry had worked in about a dozen odd jobs, typically getting fired after only a few days. He had various explanations, to which I listened with curiosity and respect without challenging their irrationality. I used LEAP: I listened reflectively, empathized, delayed giving what would have been hurtful opinions, and focused on areas where we agreed. When I finally gave my opinion, I used the three A's.

My brother wanted something from me. He wanted me to give him the pocket money he desired. He was asking for just $5 a day. I agreed to do this provided he would accept a long-acting antipsychotic medication (see Chapter 11). It took about three months of back and forth, but in the end, Henry ultimately agreed to this (despite still being certain he was not mentally ill).

And, unlike the first seven years of his illness, when he would end up in the hospital four times a year on average, over the next eighteen years he stayed on the medication and out of the hospital. Except for one time when he signed *himself* in because of anxiety!

More importantly, our relationship was back to what it was before he became ill. We again were two brothers who were very close, loved spending time together, and trusted each other.

It took some time, but eventually we agreed that when he took his medication, he stayed out of the hospital. From Henry's perspective, he stayed out because I stopped calling the police and crisis team when he took medicine. He attributed the relationship between taking his pills and not being hospitalized to a reduction in the pressure he was getting to stay on the medication rather than any benefit derived from the drugs themselves. In other words, he knew that if he stayed on the medication, his doctor and family would not force the issue of hospitalization.

My brother Henry, Matt, Vicky, and Dolores were all able to come to agreements and partner on those areas of shared common ground. Partnering is all about taking those areas of agreement, developing a plan together, and deciding to work together to reach common goals.

――

He took medications he believed he didn't need because of relationships.

――

Only two months before my brother Henry's untimely death in an accident (see Chapter 20), I told him that when I gave talks, people often asked me if he believed he had an illness and then I asked him. "Do you believe you have an illness?"

"Oh, Javi [his nickname for me]! Sure, I have schizophrenia!" he said, laughing.

"Seriously…what do you think?"

"No. I don't have a mental illness."

"Then why do you take the medicine?" I asked, genuinely curious to know what he would say.

"I do it for you and Mom and Pops." "Mom" and "Pops" were Betty and James who ran the halfway house he lived in. They were loving people who had respectful, non-judgmental relationships with my big brother.

What Henry was saying was that *he took medications he believed he didn't need because of relationships.* This was further confirmation to me of the power of relationships in helping someone with anosognosia accept treatment.

Matt

After the hospitalization I told you about in Chapter 4, Matt's parents decided to meet with me so that I could help them develop the communication skills and techniques I've been describing. As a result, they were able to form a partnership and treatment agreement with Matt that was similar to the one I made with Henry. Matt and his parents agreed that it was very important to try to keep him out of the hospital and to reduce the high level of conflict they had at home.

They abandoned the approach of confronting their son with his illness in favor of a more practical and productive approach.

The Blackburns were quick to see the benefits of LEAP. They were tired of fighting with their son and sorely needed a break from all the hostility that had built up between them over the years. They abandoned the approach of confronting Matt with his illness in favor of a more practical and productive approach — LEAP. They listened and learned that Matt wanted to stay out of the hospital as much as they wanted him to, and he also wished desperately for peace at home.

The peace emerged naturally as the Blackburns backed off from trying to convince their son he was ill. It took about two months, but Matt slowly began to listen and to understand how his parents felt about the medication he refused to take. He felt bad that his mother became frightened when he didn't take his medication.

If you recall what Matt was like at home and how he felt about taking the medication, this may sound a little farfetched. But Matt's guilt emerged from many discussions with his parents — mostly with his mother — during which they never once told him what he should do, listened reflectively, and empathized with their son's feelings. They asked questions, and when he asked them what they thought, they delayed and gave their opinion using the three A's. They especially made sure to acknowledge that they could be wrong. They didn't think it was likely they were wrong about why he needed to take medication, but they could *consider* the possibility.

Matt felt bad when his mother told him she was frightened when he stopped taking the medication. For this reason — and because his parents told him they might not be able to live with him any longer if he did *not* take the medicine — Matt agreed that the advantages to taking it far outweighed the disadvantages.

This did not happen overnight, but the result was that Matt and his parents accomplished both of the goals they had set out to achieve. A few years later, I received a holiday card from the Blackburns. Beneath Mrs. Blackburn's graceful penmanship wishing me a happy New Year, her husband had scrawled a little note:

"Thanks again for your help. We've finally got our relationship with our son back and Matt has not been in the hospital in over a year!"

Dolores

Dolores and I agreed on something similar to what the Blackburns had agreed upon—and on her goal of getting a job. As a result, I looked for opportunities to share my hypothesis that she might need to be on medication *in order to keep a job.*

Unlike my brother, but like most people with these illnesses, Dolores was nearly symptom-free when she took her medication. So, working full-time again in a demanding job was not totally out of the question—*if* she stayed on the medication consistently.

As you may recall, I asked her to keep an open mind about the possibility that medications might make it easier for her to work. At the time, she didn't think I was correct and we *agreed to disagree.* But she *did* accept my suggestion that she become a "scientist" and keep an open mind.

It took three hospitalizations and encouragement from her family and outpatient psychiatrist, but Dolores finally agreed that taking medication would very likely help her to get and keep a job and lower tensions at home.

While preparing the revision of this book, I wrote to Dolores to ask how she was doing and she answered. She graduated from college and has been working the for the past ten years. She told me she takes her medicine regularly, that it "doesn't bother" her, and that she is "so used to taking it." She does it, she says, for her family—so they feel less anxious.

At the risk of being redundant, I want to highlight a common theme in all the stories I just told you about.

The hope of repairing and sustaining relationships were critical in helping each of them accept psychiatric medication despite the fact that none believed they had a mental illness. The science supports my experience as both a family member and a clinician—relationships that are *judgment-free* and *respectful* are the key to unlocking the door to treatment.

Part III

Staying on Guard and Next Steps

"Hope is a good thing—maybe the best thing—
and no good thing ever dies."
—Stephen King—

"Love many things, for therein lies the true strength, and whosoever
loves much performs much, and can accomplish much, and what is
done in love is done well."
—Vincent van Gogh—

10

Don't Let Your Guard Down: The problem of poor adherence

I have, as I've said, used LEAP to convince patients to accept medication on a trial basis, even though they continued to believe they were not ill. But I have also learned the hard way always to remember that this person still believes there's nothing wrong with him, and that his belief often leads to his "accidentally," or unconsciously, missing doses. However, if you also consider the fact that people who are not mentally ill but need to take medication (for any number of serious medical problems) also have trouble remembering to take their medicine[1], you will see how many doses are likely to be missed.

The problems that arise from such "partial-compliance" can be more subtle, but no less significant, than what happens when someone stops taking his medication completely. For one thing, if everyone (doctor and family) believes the patient is taking his medication regularly and it doesn't appear to be working, they'll assume it's been given a fair trial when that is far from the truth. I've seen many medications written off as ineffective for a particular individual because no one knew the person was

---

1 Often, people simply forget to take their medicine. Medication adherence rates in other medical illnesses range from 15 to 50%.

missing many, but not all, doses. But even if the medicine appears to have some—but not enough—benefit, the doctor may be afraid to raise a high dose even higher when, in fact, the patient is not taking the entire dose prescribed in the first place!

How do I know all this? First, from my experience conducting thousands of interviews using LEAP. I have heard many "confessions" of skipped doses. When someone trusts that you will not scold, criticize, or even comment on such admissions, they feel freer to share them. Add to that the empathy and normalization that follows when you use LEAP (e.g., "I would have skipped the dose too if it were me."), and you are more likely to hear the truth in the future.

But research also shows that poor compliance rates (complete and partial non-adherence) average between 50 and 75%. Psychiatrists have been found to dramatically overestimate the rate of compliance in their patients. I think they should be forgiven—because if their patients were anything like my brother Henry, they are telling their doctors what they want to hear.

The stark fact remains that only 25% of our patients are taking their medication as prescribed. So what can be done to engage such patients in treatment and give them the tools to remember to take all their medication as prescribed?

11

Medications

The message light on my answering machine was blinking. I hit the play button and heard, "Xavier, I am calling because Henry missed his appointment for his Prolixin injection today. Please ask him to give me a call to reschedule."[1] It was my brother's case manager, Patricia. Henry and I had met with her after his last hospitalization and agreed that she would be allowed to call me if he missed one of his appointments. It was 1989, and in the past twelve months, Henry had not been admitted to the hospital even once, whereas in the past he had been in and out of psychiatric hospitals about four times a year. I believe now, as I did then, that he had done so much better for several reasons — the therapist he was working with, the change in the way I was talking to him (see Chapter 6: Listen), and especially, the way in which he was now getting his medicine.

During his last hospitalization, I had lobbied hard to convince Henry to try a long-acting injectable (LAI) medication, rather than taking pills orally, because over the years as a clinician working in hospitals I had seen how much it helped so many others who had

---

1 Long-acting injectable Prolixin (generic name: Fluphenazine Decanoate) is one of three such antipsychotic medicines, all of which last approximately two weeks per injection. The other two are Haldol and Risperdal CONSTA. Haldol and Prolixin are among the older, 1st generation antipsychotic medications and Risperdal is one of the newer 2nd generation antipsychotic medications, also called "atypical antipsychotics." There are several more long-acting antipsychotic medications available today.

also been labeled "revolving-door" patients (or "frequent flyers"). At that time, long-acting injectable, or depo, medicines were typically prescribed to individuals being treated involuntarily in the hospital. The rationale was simple: This person has a history of not believing he is ill and he stops taking his medicine when he leaves the hospital. Consequently, we'll give him something that will last for two weeks at a time. And if he stops taking the medicine (i.e., misses an appointment for the injection), we will know and will be able to reach out to him.

Long-acting injectable medications should be among the first line drug treatments.

For too long LAI medications have been considered a treatment of last resort. They are offered only after all other avenues have failed. Both the research and my experience tell me that the opposite is true. For patients like my brother, who had longstanding problems with insight—and for many others who have difficulty with partial adherence—LAI medications should be among the first line drug treatments. In other words, they should be among the first medications offered to someone diagnosed with a psychotic disorder.

I have seen this strategy work time and again. It's common sense when you think about it. Before Henry agreed to the injections, he would typically promise that if he were released from the hospital, he would continue to take his medicine. In fact, he did just what any of us would have done if we believed we'd been wrongfully forced into a hospital and treated for an illness we didn't believe we had. We would tell the doctors and our worried family members what they wanted to hear. "I see now that I am sick and need to take the medicine." It's common sense.

Nevertheless, having to be dishonest with loved ones who are pushing you to take medicine and allying themselves with the psychiatrists who are convinced you are "crazy" is a terrible and lonely predicament to be in.

Before I learned how to listen to my brother, I was angry and felt betrayed whenever he reneged on his promise. But after learning what it was like for him to have to hide pills and lie, after hearing how humiliated and bad he felt about being dishonest, I wanted to find a way to avoid putting him in that predicament.

A simple solution was to lay everything out on the table and not create a situation in which he would be tempted to secretly stop taking the medicine. That is one of several reasons long-acting injectable medication was so helpful to him. All he had to do was show up for an appointment every two weeks and meet with someone he liked. The brief prick of the needle twice a month[2] was far less difficult for him than having to struggle three times a day with the conflict between loyalty to his family and his desire to stop taking the medicine. He wanted to please our mother and me because he knew how worried we were about him, but because his illness had convinced him nothing was wrong, he found himself caught between a rock and a hard place more than 90 times a month! Now it was just twice a month, and we all knew whenever the conflict got the best of him and the "denial" won out.

Another similar case with which I am personally familiar involved Millie, who is the mother of Tina and Susan and the subject of Susan's documentary film "Out of the Shadow" (see Resources section at the back of this book). I was the consultant for the film and am also a family friend. Like my brother, Millie has a long history of schizophrenia and of hiding the fact that she is not taking her medicine. Once, while flying on an airplane on her way to visit Susan, Millie went into the bathroom, poured out the contents of every one of her capsules of antipsychotic

---

2 New formulations of 2nd generation LAI's have been developed that need to be given only once a month and even once every three months.

medication, then put the empty capsules back together and into the bottle. She did this because she knew her daughter would be checking to see if she was swallowing the pills. I can't blame Millie for what she did — she didn't think she was ill. I wouldn't want to take medicine for an illness I didn't believe I had! Would you? I would probably do the same thing if I were in her shoes.

As the film shows, when Millie is taking her medication, she does wonderfully, but she relapses whenever she is able to avoid taking the medicine. It was during her last relapse, when Susan and Tina were talking together with me about Millie's treatment options, that I strongly encouraged them to get her on Risperdal CONSTA. She had previously done well on atypical medications, and I felt that a long-acting injectable would give Millie the best chance of staying well and recovering more fully. At that time, and as of this writing, CONSTA was the only atypical antipsychotic available in a long-acting injectable form. Susan and Tina were able to use their positive relationship with their mother to convince her to accept twice-monthly injections, and, not surprisingly, since she has been on this form of medication there has not been another relapse (to my knowledge). Among other positive benefits, Millie is no longer tempted to secretly stop taking her pills and is now on a steady dose of medication, unable to act on her natural ambivalence without her doctor and family knowing about it.

Medication: Which One and How It's Given

Very often, when I'm giving a LEAP seminar, someone wants to know, "What medication is best?" The answer is "none." My experience and the science agree that we cannot reliably predict which medication will be best for any particular individual. When deciding on a specific medication one needs to balance, among other things, how well it is working against the side effects for that individual. In some instances, cost is also a deciding factor.

That said, however, I believe that certain generalizations can be made when it comes to choosing medications for people with a history of poor insight and poor adherence to medication. In short, keep the dosing simple and make it hard for the person to succumb to his desire to stop taking the medicine.

My advice is to keep it simple if you can.

When a medication is taken once or twice a day as compared to several times a day or more, it is far easier to monitor the patient's adherence. And it is also easier for the person taking the medicine to remember and not succumb to an unconscious desire to skip a dose. The fewer doses per day, the fewer opportunities the person will have to consciously or unconsciously decide to skip a dose. Or simply to forget.

When patients of mine have a history of poor insight and poor adherence to medication, I often recommend a long-acting injectable drug.

When patients of mine have a history of poor insight and poor adherence (i.e., partial or complete non-compliance) to medication, I often recommend a long-acting injectable drug. Not only does this make it easier for the patient and easier for me to monitor his compliance, but it does away with other issues as well. For example, the person administering the dose doesn't have to ask the patient to open his mouth to prove he swallowed the pills (I would be thrilled if I never had to do that again) or secretly count how many pills are left in the bottle to try and get a read on whether or not he is taking all his medicine.

But once again, you do not have to take my word for it (nor would I want you to). Research supports what I've learned from personal experience. For example, in 1999, Young and his colleagues published a comprehensive review of research studies (see literature cited at the back of this book) that found that, on average, about 50% of the patients taking pills stopped taking their medication as compared to only 17% of those who were receiving long-acting injections. This essential finding has been replicated numerous times. If you decide to go this route, don't be scared off by the prospect of trying to convince someone to take a shot twice a month. It's not as difficult as you might think. In fact, I have been involved in some research on this issue[3] and found that if you use the main elements of LEAP, you are likely to be successful. But whether or not you can convince the person you are trying to help to take a long-acting injectable medication, remember to simplify the dosing, closely monitor that the medicine is actually being taken, and never stop listening to how your patient or loved one experiences taking medicine.

As a final comment on the subject of medication, I'd like to speak to a question I'm frequently asked: "If anosognosia is a symptom of mental illness, like flat affect or hallucinations, can medicines help?"

As I've already said, few studies have examined this question specifically. Generally, anosognosia, like other negative symptoms, appears to be resistant to drug treatment. Although two studies in the literature suggest that Clozaril and Risperdal CONSTA may improve insight,[4] it's important to remember the importance of replication (i.e., Aristotle's observation that "one swallow does not make a summer"). These studies, though

3 Lasser R, Gharabawi GM, Jarboe K, Litrell K, Miller AL, M.D., Amador XF, Weiden PJ,Schooler NR, Docherty JP, and Crumbley E. (2005). Patient Acceptance and Long-Acting Risperidone: the Start Program and Gain Approach. Presentation at the annual meeting of the American Psychiatric Association.

4 Study 1: Pallanti S, Quercioli L, Pazzagli A (1999), Effects of clozapine on awareness of illness and cognition in schizophrenia. *Psychiatry Res* 86(3):239-249. Study 2: Paillot C, Goetz R, and Amador XF. Double blind, randomized, controlled study of a psychotherapy [LEAP] designed to improve motivation for change, insight into schizophrenia and adherence to medication (Abstract). *Schizophrenia Bulletin*, 35 (Supp. 1): 343, 2009.

promising, must be independently replicated before we can know if the findings are valid.

Psychotherapy

Does psychotherapy do anything for people with serious mental illness? If you've read this far, you now know why I believe it does. Many people have asked me for referrals to therapists who use LEAP. Others have asked me for advice about how to convince a therapist who is not trained in LEAP to try this method.

Since the first edition of this book was published in the summer of 2000, tens of thousands of therapists and family members have been trained in LEAP. LEAP is as much a communication style as it is a form of therapy and, because it is intuitive and helps very quickly, most therapists are willing to learn it once they get a feel for it.

Many therapists already use some elements of LEAP,
but not as systematically as they should and without
understanding its full potential.

It has been my experience that many therapists already use some elements of LEAP, but not as systematically as they should and without understanding its full potential. When I point out the specific instances when they have used reflective listening, the cornerstone of this method of communicating with patients, they quickly acknowledge that it reduces tension and distrust and opens lines of honest communication about symptoms and treatment. At its best, it helps patients find reasons to be in treatment that make sense to them and transforms the LEAP practitioner from a potential adversary into someone patients trust and whose opinion they value. For these reasons, I find that once they get a taste of it, most therapists are not only open but eager to learn more about this way of working.

Many therapists have been trained in LEAP through LEAP Institute (see *www.LEAPInstitute.org*). We have only recently begun to compile a list of certified therapists, however thousands of others have attended LEAP trainings over the past decade that we have not kept track of. So, if you cannot find a certified LEAP trained therapist in your community, there are some questions you can ask to find out if the therapist you are dealing with or considering has attended one of our earlier seminars and is using the core LEAP tools. For example, you can ask if he or she has ever attended a LEAP seminar or training day or read this book. You can ask if they've seen Dr. Amador's TED Talk. You can ask if he or she has received any training in Motivational Interviewing. If the answer to any or all is "no," you can then ask if he or she would be willing to read this book and lend them your copy.

How to Convince a Therapist to Read this Book

While it's somewhat embarrassing for me to offer this next bit of advice and run the risk of offending my fellow therapists, I do it because I've been told countless times by readers who are family members, "We gave a copy of your book to our loved one's therapist, but we don't think he's read it! How do we get him to read it?"

I have contemplated this question, wondering what I would do if I were that therapist. And then I've remembered that on occasion, I have, indeed, been given books by patients and family members. One of the things that usually got me to crack the book's spine was a request for my opinion—questions like "I thought this book was helpful and I'd like to work this way; what do you think? Should I?" usually got me to read at least the first chapter and skim the rest. You could try questions such as, "Our family has been working this way with our loved one and we wanted to make sure we weren't interfering with anything you're doing. Could you have a quick look and let us know?"

Don't be discouraged if you encounter some initial resistance. Remember that it took me seven years of arguing with my brother before I started to work this way! And, in fact, most therapists got into the business because they have a genuine desire to be helpful.

Cognitive Therapy

Finally, cognitive therapy has proven to be effective for reducing the severity of certain symptoms in patients with psychotic disorders (See Chapter 17 on Psychotherapy for Psychosis). As I mentioned earlier, the fact that we are dealing with disorders of the brain means that we need to attack the deficits with both biological and psychological treatments, just as we do when someone has a stroke or some other form of brain dysfunction.

Despite being effective for many patients, however, cognitive therapy is still underutilized in the treatment of psychotic disorders in the U.S., whereas in other countries, such as the United Kingdom, it is more widely available. Nevertheless, its use is growing. I devote a chapter to this topic and, at the end of this book, I provide you with recommended readings and an organizational resource so that you can learn more about this important tool for the treatment of psychosis.

Having said all this, however, there are times when we can't wait for LEAP or other forms of psychotherapy to take effect. If someone is off medication and in crisis, we may need to step in and take over. Doing that is rarely easy. In the next three chapters, I'll help you recognize when it's time to seek involuntary treatment and how to go about it. But just as importantly, I'll explain how you can use LEAP to preserve your relationship with your loved one, even when you need to take these drastic measures.

12

Involuntary Treatment

When I give lectures and workshops on LEAP, I am often applauded as someone who has helped both those who would like to see more options for involuntary treatment and those who would like to have such laws revoked. The first edition of *I Am Not Sick, I Don't Need Help!* has been used by some people to argue that less intrusive measures, such as LEAP, are available and should be used in place of involuntary treatment, while others point to the research on anosognosia to argue that involuntary treatment is the humane thing to do when someone refuses treatment because of poor insight.

So, where do I stand on this issue?

We need these laws, but when or whether they should be invoked depends on individual circumstances. I have personally been involved in initiating more involuntary treatments than I can count. I have no doubt that my participation in such treatments not only saved lives but also helped my patients avoid injury or being arrested and charged with a crime. Certainly, the interventions gave many a shot at recovery from mental illness.

But for me, involuntary treatment is often the last resort. For all those it has helped, I know that many times it was traumatic for the person with mental illness and little more than a band-aid (unless the ordered treatment was continued on an outpatient basis).

Over the years, I have learned a lot about when and how to pursue this option and how to optimize the outcome. It does not have to be a traumatic experience for your loved one or for you. In this chapter, I will talk about those instances when I believe forcing treatment is necessary, the options available to you, and some advice on how to do it.

Certain situations are a "no-brainer" and almost always warrant commitment.

In Chapter 1, I described how Matt's mother called the police when Matt became threatening during an argument because she knew from past experience that he was losing control of his temper and would likely become violent. Having survived many episodes of her son's illness, she knew when it was time to call for help.

On the face of it, the signs of illness to which Matt's mother was alert were different from those I learned to watch for in my brother Henry. But the degree of danger they signaled was very similar. The signs for which you need to learn to watch may also be unique. But whenever a person is acting in a threatening or dangerous manner either verbally (e.g., "Stop transmitting waves at me or I will make you stop!" or more blatantly (e.g., "I am going to hit you if…" or "I am going to kill you…") or physically (e.g., throwing things, pushing or restraining another person, lighting a fire in a waste basket, picking up a bat or knife, locking you out of the house or locking you in a room, etc.), you have to act. The same holds true if the person is expressing any ideas about ending his own life. Certain situations are "no-brainers" and almost always warrant commitment. Obvious among these are those situations in which someone is obviously about to hurt himself or someone else. In fact, being harmful to oneself or others is the most common legal standard for committing someone to a hospital against his will.

If you are the doctor or therapist, it is almost always good practice to contact the family to share your observations and concerns.

If you have decided to act, remember that you are not the first person who has had to commit a mentally ill person and there are many resources available to you. If you are a family member, the first person to contact when you feel the situation is spiraling out of control is the therapist or doctor who has been working with your loved one (if he or she is seeing someone). If he has not seen a therapist or doctor in a long time, or has never seen a mental health professional, the first person you contact will have to be someone different, and I will get to that shortly.

If you are a doctor or therapist, it is almost always good practice to contact the family to share your observations and concerns. Hopefully, you have been working as a team up to this point. But even if you haven't, it's never too late to join forces. For many therapists, this advice goes against their training and ethics. What is said in therapy is supposed to stay in the room, with very few exceptions. But, although most therapists are not currently trained this way, an exacerbation of a serious mental illness (e.g., psychotic decompensation) is good cause to breach confidentiality so that you can speak with others who care about your patient. If the limits of confidentiality are clear up front ("If you become sick and it affects your good judgment, I will need to inform your family to get their help"), there is no ethical dilemma. I have done this many times and have never been sued or received complaints. More importantly, it's the right thing to do.

How to Proceed with Involuntary Treatment

There are generally three ways to start the ball rolling. So far, I have only mentioned calling the police. In fact, there are other options I almost always consider first unless I feel someone is clearly in immediate danger of harming himself or someone else. Ideally, my order of preference is to: 1) Go together to the ER; 2) Call a mental health crisis team or an assertive community treatment team; or if all else fails, 3) Call the police and ask for officers from the department's Crisis Intervention Team (CIT).[1]

My order of preference is to:

1.   *Go together to the E.R.*
2.   *Call a mental health crisis team or assertive community treatment team*
3.   *Call the police and ask for officers from the department's Crisis Intervention Team (CIT)*

Use Your Leap Skills to Make This Happen

Sometimes, if your relationship is one in which the person still trusts you, you can ask him to go to the ER with you. Explain that you're worried about him and want to see if the doctor can help. Use your LEAP skills to make this happen. And be sure to focus on what the person believes the problem to be. Once, when Henry was very ill and paranoid about our mother, believing she would kill him, I said, "You need to get away from Mom right now. Let's go for a ride and drop by Kino [the county hospital] so you can feel safer." He agreed. One mother convinced her mentally ill daughter to go to the hospital with her after they had talked about the daughter's suicidal feelings. The mother, after doing reflective listening and normalizing her daughter's feelings

---

1 CIT is another fast growing innovative and effective approach to helping persons with mental illness. For more information please see: (http://www.citinternational.org/).

about wanting to die, then asked, "Can I tell you what I would do if I were you?"

"What do you think I should do?"

"I think we should go together and talk to a doctor just in case that helps. And if you still feel this way afterwards, then you haven't really lost anything."

"But they'll lock me up if I go."

"They might. But even if they do, you don't have anything to lose. If you still feel this way later, at least you will know that you tried." By using reflective listening and not lying about what was likely to happen, she was able to convince her daughter to go to the hospital.

You may be tempted, but try hard not to trick the person by telling him you are going someplace else and then ending up at the ER. I know many people who have tried this trick, and I did it myself once, but it's risky for two reasons: The person will justifiably feel betrayed and/or might jump out of the car when he realizes where you are really going. It can work, but I don't recommend it over the other options.

To find out if your community has a crisis team, you can call any psychiatric emergency room or your local police department.

Many police departments and psychiatric emergency rooms work in partnership to keep mentally ill people who commit minor offenses (such as disturbing the peace) out of jail. A common product of this partnership is the "mobile crisis team" (a.k.a. crisis team, mobile acute crisis team, psychiatric crisis unit, etc.). Usually, mobile crisis teams are based in mental health agencies or hospitals. To find out if your community has a crisis team, you can call any psychiatric emergency room or your local police department.

The way this type of intervention works is that the mental health workers come to your loved one and evaluate him on the spot. If they judge that hospitalization is warranted, they will try to convince your loved one to accompany them to the hospital. If he refuses, they can initiate the commitment process immediately. Because they're trained to recognize mental illness, they're less apt than the police to misinterpret your loved one's behavior as something else (e.g., criminal behavior, the result of a negative character trait, etc.). They may also be able to communicate with your loved one more effectively than the average police officer who has not received the same specialized training. If no mobile crisis team exists, or none is unavailable when you call, then contact your local police. When you do, explain that your loved one is mentally ill and in imminent danger of hurting himself or someone else (if applicable).

You may naturally be resistant to the idea of calling the police because you feel that by having your loved one committed, you are trying to take control of his life. And, if you are already struggling with a tenuous or strained relationship, it is only natural to want to avoid the conflict such a move will create.

This avoidance and the desire to not be hurtful often lead to procrastination and second thoughts. This is normal but potentially dangerous for all the reasons I discussed in Chapter 2 (i.e., poor response to treatment when left untreated for years, poorer course of illness, suicide, risk of violence, etc.). It is also dangerous because so many people with untreated mental illness end up in our jails and prisons.

This is not a good solution — our jails and prisons are notorious for providing inadequate mental health treatment. Worse, the individual who has been charged and jailed usually ends up with a criminal record that will forever change the course of his life. In tens of thousands of cases, such persons lose a lot more than 72 hours (the typical involuntary treatment hold) of their freedom. If you initiate an involuntary treatment the chances of this happening are far less than when a complete stranger is the triggering cause. But to succeed, it is imperative for you to believe that commitment is not a permanent violation of your loved one's autonomy. In fact, in most cases it is a means by which you can help your loved one regain control of his life and self-determination. That is why resolving your ambivalence and guilt early on is vital to the commitment process.

Resolving your ambivalence and guilt

As right as you think your decision is, it's difficult not to feel guilty sometimes and to falter in your resolve. The term "commitment" conjures up images of physical struggle and straitjackets. When we think of a psychiatric ward, the picture of a nurturing and stabilizing environment is generally not the one that comes to mind. Images from the movie *One Flew Over the Cuckoo's Nest* are far more common.

Like most people, I initially had a very negative image of psychiatric institutions. I wrote in my preface to the first edition of this book:

> "Having never stepped foot inside a psychiatric ward, I felt nervous and self-conscious. Nervous for the same reasons most people are made uneasy when surrounded by twenty or so people with serious mental illness. Some of them were pacing and talking aloud to the voices they alone heard. Others were passionately smoking cigarettes. One man sat quietly, directly in front of me, his eyes fixed on some far away vision. Was I safe? Were they safe? Was this a hell-hole or a haven? These were just a few of the anxious questions running through my mind…I was sure I would somehow be blamed for what had happened to my brother… for the police, the ambulance, and the restraints he had endured because of me."

In fact, after my brother was committed the first time, I learned that the ward he went to was nothing like what I imagined in my worst fears. Yes, there was a lot of smoking (although even that is now a thing of the past), but no one was sitting around in straitjackets screaming. None of the patients were threatening or bothered me in any way. Henry had been restrained, but that had been only briefly and in the ambulance. When he got to the ER, they soon released him from the lambskin-lined cuffs. The ward he was on, like many I have worked in, had a day room or lounge, with a television playing softly in one corner. There was a ping-pong table on the other side of the room. I was able to visit my brother and spend time with him in that room. The reality of the ward quickly allayed my worst fears.

The truth is that most in-patient treatment facilities are designed to be comfortable, humane, and reassuring to the people who are being treated there.

In order to effectively help your loved one, it is necessary to either work through, or temporarily put aside, the fears and doubts you have about commitment. The most important thing you need to do is try to separate myth from reality. Learn about the commitment process and what the facilities in your area are like. Many of the consumer-based (or patient-based) organizations described in the Resources section of this book can help you to learn what you can expect from your local mental health facilities.

This advice is relevant for some mental health professionals as well. So many times, those of us who work primarily in outpatient settings hesitate to commit patients because of a fear of facilities with which we are not intimately familiar.

Serious mental illness is like any other medical illness. If your loved one had diabetes, you would learn everything you could about the illness and what steps to take to control the disease. You would try to locate the best centers for the treatment of diabetes in your area. You would have emergency medical numbers by the phone and know the closest emergency facility in case anything unexpected happened. If the diabetes flared up and your loved one became confused and disoriented, you would not hesitate to pursue hospitalization, whether your loved one wanted it or not. And I am fairly certain that you would not feel guilty or ambivalent.

Serious mental illness is like any other medical illness.

Recognize the Warning Signs

If you have gone through previous hospitalizations with your loved one, you are probably familiar with the early warning signs that signal the need for hospitalization. You know when your loved one is acting out of character and the illness has worsened. Take a moment to stop and write down the three most worrisome changes in your loved one's thinking, perceptions, and/or actions that you feel warranted hospitalization in the past (or that you think should warrant it).

1.

2.

3.

Keep your list in mind and refer to it often. If you are mindful of the early warning signs, you will be less likely to get caught off guard when the illness flares up. Here are some common signs that others have considered serious enough for them to contemplate commitment:

- Refuses to take medication when the family and therapist know from past experience that deterioration and harm are imminent
- Verbally or physically abusive
- Suicidal ideas (e.g., "I wish I was dead," "I should just end it all," etc.)
- Harms self (e.g., cuts body parts, bangs head, drinks soap, eats dirt, etc.)
- Is destructive of property (own or others)
- Stalks others (e.g., incessant phone calls despite complaints, repeated unwanted visits, etc.)
- Homeless, resulting in harm to self (e.g., exposure to extreme weather conditions without appropriate clothing, poor nutrition, neglect of essential health care, etc.)
- Refuses or is unable to speak with anyone
- Delusions of grandeur (e.g., has superhuman powers, is famous, knows famous people personally, etc.)
- Talks to self excessively
- Speech is unintelligible
- Delusions of persecution (e.g., being watched by government agents, possessed by the devil, fears loved ones intend harm, etc.)
- Command hallucinations (e.g., voices that say "you must kill yourself," etc.)
- Significant deterioration in self-care and hygiene
- Dangerous due to disorganization (e.g., starts fires unintentionally by dropping lit cigarettes, etc.)

- Inadequate care of dependents (e.g., neglect, isolates children or the elderly from other family members, etc.)
- Poor judgment (e.g., uncharacteristically sexually provocative and/or promiscuous, stops paying bills, wild spending sprees, gives away all possessions, loses job due to "eccentric" behavior, fails to keep appointments, or fails to follow procedures necessary to receive benefits)
- Health is deteriorating (e.g., self starvation, refuses to seek medical help for other serious illnesses, mixes prescribed medications with illicit drugs, etc.)

These examples may or may not be relevant to your situation. I list them for two reasons: to give you an idea of what others have found to be important signs and to remind you that you are not the only person who has had to make this decision. In the Resources section you will find a list of organizations that can put you in touch with people who have had firsthand experience dealing with commitments (e.g., www.nami.org, www.psychlaws.org, and others).

There are less immediate methods: the civil commitment hearing and court-ordered assisted outpatient treatment.

In addition to the three avenues just described, there are several less immediate methods: the civil commitment hearing, guardianship, advance directives (where the person with mental illness, when doing well, has legally designated someone to take charge of his treatment should he become ill again), and court-ordered assisted outpatient treatment (AOT). Since the first edition of this book was published, more options for AOT have been created in a number of states across America. Although inpatient involuntary treatment typically requires that the mental illness make the person a danger to self or others, persons with chronic psychotic disorders who show certain patterns of behavior as a consequence of their illness may receive court-ordered treatment on an outpatient basis. To find out if your state has such a law and how to use it, I encourage you to go to the Treatment Advocacy Center's website, *www.psychlaws.org*. There, you will also find information on guardianship, advance directives, and other options.

The Treatment Advocacy Center is funded by the Stanley Research Foundation and was founded by psychiatrist E. Fuller Torrey and others who were concerned about the millions of mentally ill Americans who were refusing treatment because of anosognosia (poor insight) and suffering terribly as a result.

Remember Michael Kass, from Chapter 4, the patient I met in the ER? He had been found hiding in a subway train tunnel. When the police found him, he hadn't eaten or bathed in several days and he had made camp dangerously close to an active track, explaining that "they [federal agents] would never think to look for me here."

Michael had a history of responding well to medication. When he was on medicine, he was able to care for himself and did not do things that put his life in danger. But because he didn't see that he was ill, he always stopped taking the medicine the moment he was discharged from the hospital, thus starting the cycle all over again. Michael is one of the many people who have benefited from AOT.

He understood that I believed I was helping him, even though he didn't agree that he needed help.

When you commit someone to a hospital you may feel that you have created an irreparable breach of trust. But when it's done from a position of love and support, it is almost always perceived positively. From my personal experience with my brother, I know that (although it took about four hospitalizations) Henry eventually came to see my interventions into his life (calling the police and his psychiatrists) as expressions of my love for him. He understood that I believed I was helping him, even though he didn't agree that he needed help. This was a great source of consolation for both of us during the next several years it took for him to realize that he was in need of treatment (i.e., for us to agree).

In this chapter, we've talked about how to determine whether and when to commit. Since you chose to read it, the answer may be that the time to commit is now. If, after using the techniques I've offered, your loved one is still refusing treatment, you have probably begun to seriously consider commitment as an option. If your loved one is seriously ill and not getting treatment, he or she needs help now. Remember that if this same person were suffering from a flare-up of some other medical condition like diabetes or had been in an accident, you would not hesitate to corral him into the car and take him to the hospital, no matter how much he protested. Sooner or later, even if he still believes he is not sick, if you can help him to recognize that what you did was done out of love, he will most likely be grateful.

13

How to Do It

I was 21 years old and deciding on a career in psychology when schizophrenia exploded in Henry's brain like some impossibly patient time bomb planted by his genes. Suddenly, only a day after our stepfather's death, Henry was talking about hearing voices and having "crazy" thoughts that couldn't possibly be true. He was 29 at the time but had been slowly becoming odd and isolated since his mid-twenties.

The night our stepfather died of a heart attack, it was Henry who found him on the high school track where Dad had gone jogging. I was the first one Henry called with the news. I called my older brothers and sisters who lived scattered across the country and left that same night for Arizona, where Henry was living with our parents. The next morning, Henry met me at the airport.

During the half-hour drive across town in his bright blue '52 Chevy pickup, I struggled with feeling embarrassed whenever we had to stop at a red light, but not because of the thirty-year-old truck painted the color of a turquoise Caribbean sea. True, the color was strange even for Tucson in the early eighties and caused a few stoplight stares, but Henry's choice of color didn't embarrass me. As far as I was concerned, Henry could paint that truck any color under the sun after all the blood and sweat he poured into its resurrection. Damned thing could have been pink, and I would still think of Henry as a model of masculinity. He must have rebuilt motors on a dozen cars in his day.

No, I could never be embarrassed by his bright blue pick-up. It was the talking to himself that made me wonder what we must have looked like to other drivers. Henry wasn't looking at me. Maybe he couldn't. Mostly he stared straight ahead, talking and laughing to himself. Sometimes, he would turn to look out his open window at the car next to us and just keep on talking nonsense to the passenger in the adjacent car. At every stoplight, I saw perplexed and fearful expressions, a window rolled up, at one, "the finger."

Green lights offered some relief from the tension that was building inside me; no one would notice now, and it was just the two of us. Or was it? Henry kept right on talking and mumbling to himself as if I weren't there, almost as if he were having a conversation with someone I couldn't see. When I first asked him what he was saying, he laughed and said, "Ohh, Javi my little brother, he's here, ha ha ha." Then, abruptly becoming serious, "Dad had an accident. Oh, no, no, no. I was playing the guitar when I killed him, the music got in his head and he tripped and fell, he was too, he mmmhuh bad Papi his soul you know? His bow-toe-blow you know?" His speech kept dissolving like that into unintelligible syllables and nonsensical rhymes mumbled over an occasional phrase. Mostly word salad, with fragments of coherent thoughts — disturbing thoughts. After a few more attempts at rational conversation, I gave up. I was still processing the news he had given me over the phone the night before. As odd as my brother sounded — I was playing the guitar when I killed him — I was mostly thinking of my mother, who had just lost her second husband, and about myself. I was not yet concerned about what was happening to Henry.

By the time Henry and I arrived at my parents' house, now my mother's house, I had successfully tuned him out. But over the course of that longest day of my young life, it became clear to me that he was very seriously sick. He was psychotic. Maybe even schizophrenic. Most people, including my family at the time, don't know what that means. But I did. I was a senior in college, studying psychology, and I recognized the symptoms, among them hearing voices and delusions. And so by the end of that week, because I was the "family psychologist" and also the one closest to Henry, I was elected — given the task of getting Henry into the hospital or, more to the point, away from the rest of us who were grieving and reeling from our stepfather's unexpected death at the age of fifty-eight. We had a funeral to plan, a loved one to bury, and no interest in dealing with Henry's mental illness.

At first I tried to convince him he was sick and needed help, and as you well know, utterly failed. Unfortunately, being new to all this, I immediately jumped to trying to get him involuntarily committed. But the psychiatrist in the ER with whom I spoke wasn't having it. He asked me, "Is he threatening anyone?"

"No," I answered truthfully.

"Is he threatening to kill himself?"

"No."

"Then there's nothing I can do. Call back if he becomes a danger to himself or others."

Henry and I went round and round that week, but when I went back to New York he was still in the throes of his first psychotic episode. About a month later, after the rest of the family had cleared out, I received the first of many such phone calls from my mother. "You need to come here quick. Henry is not in his right mind. He needs to be in the hospital."

I returned to Arizona, and this time I was more successful. Henry had been talking about suicide. I called the police, told them he was mentally ill and suicidal, and they took him to the hospital. He was back in three hours! He was angry, hurt, and felt betrayed. "How could you call the police on your own brother? Did I steal from you? Did I try and hurt you?" Worse than that, he felt vindicated. "See! There's nothing wrong with me. Even the psychiatrist said so!"

Actually, what had happened is that Henry quickly figured out that his talking about feeling suicidal was what had triggered the police taking him into custody. He realized that as long as he didn't talk about it, he would not be admitted to the hospital. And he was right.

As we talked long into that night, I realized I had to try again. Without telling Henry what I was going to do, I called the police the very next night. I told them he was mentally ill and threatening suicide. He was also drinking too much, but I didn't add this fact. When they arrived, I stayed locked up in the bedroom with my mother so that Henry would have to answer the door. That was one of many mistakes I made that night. Fortunately, Henry went quietly, but the damage I did to our relationship took a long time to heal.

Although I was mostly well intentioned, I made many mistakes I now wish I hadn't. Some of what I did was positive, like talking to the psychiatrist after Henry was released the first time I tried to get him hospitalized. But still, I made some serious mistakes that will be instructive to talk about here.

What I Should Have Done

The first mistake I made was not encouraging Henry to talk with his therapist. He had seen a therapist the year before for depression, and although I knew that, I did not try to utilize their existing relationship. I knew Henry liked Roy, and I should have called him for advice. Ideally, I could have suggested to Henry that he meet with Roy to talk about Dad's passing and just dropped the whole "you're mentally ill and need to go to the hospital" issue.

But I wasn't thinking about Henry's perspective yet. I was being the family shrink.

After deciding to go the route of an involuntary admission to the hospital, I should first have checked to see if there was a crisis team, staffed by mental health professionals, that could come out to the house and evaluate my brother. Instead, I went straight to 911.

Before I go further, I want to be very clear that I am not being hard on myself. I was new to all this. You should not be hard on yourself either. The only time I felt guilty about my relationship with Henry was when I didn't learn from my mistakes.

The most obvious (and frankly, frightening) mistake I made was letting Henry answer the door when the police came that second time. He was psychotic, paranoid. Although more and more police are now being trained to deal with mentally ill people, back then it was very rare. A terrible tragedy could have unfolded that night if Henry had become frightened and began speaking delusionally and in a threatening manner to the officers. Had they felt they were in danger, they would have ordered him to the ground, and he, very likely, would not have been able to comply because he was so disorganized and barely in touch with reality.

Instead, I should have met the officers outside and explained that my brother was mentally ill, had no criminal history, and was not threatening to hurt anyone but himself. By saying these things I would have made it clear that they were going to meet someone who was loved and that I was asking them to take great care. But I did neither of those things. I was very lucky that night.

Finally, I should have telephoned the psychiatrist when Henry arrived at the ER so that he wouldn't again deny being suicidal and so be released. Better yet, I should have gone down in person. But again I was lucky — Henry was so upset about opening the door to find several police officers wanting to "arrest" him that, when he spoke to the psychiatrist, he apparently didn't think to hide the fact that he had been feeling suicidal.

Once Henry was admitted to the hospital, I made the very common mistake I talked about in Chapter 2. Exhausted by the whole experience, I took a break and did not stay involved.

The system is set up to put a wall between mental health professionals and their patients' families.

Although I went to a family meeting and visited my brother (he refused to speak to me during these visits), I did not attempt to stay in touch with his treatment team or participate in the discharge plan. Part of the reason was naiveté on my part and part of the reason is that the system is set up to put a wall between mental health professionals and their patients' families.

One of the most important things family members can do is to stay active and in touch with their loved one's mental health care providers. This is true whether your loved one is in the hospital or an outpatient seeing his therapist once every several weeks or more. During our one meeting with Henry's doctor and social worker, my mother and I should have asked about the discharge plan and shared our observations about what we thought would and would not work. The most important observation we could have shared is that Henry did not think he was sick. We should have held the professionals accountable with the question: "Given that he does not believe he's ill, what good will your prescription and outpatient appointment slip do?"

Henry agreed to renew his relationship with Roy, his previous therapist. But once again, I did not attempt to open a line of active communication with the therapist. For example, I did not ask Henry if I could go to his first session to explain my view of the events that had led to his hospitalization. Within days of leaving the hospital, Henry had stopped taking the medicine, and within weeks, he apparently stopped going to see Roy. I wasn't sure about the latter because I was not communicating with Roy and had to rely solely on what Henry told me. In his defense, at that time, my brother mostly wanted me to stop intruding on his life and telling him he was sick. Giving me permission to talk to his therapist was probably not going to be high on his list of priorities. But the point is I never tried.

I did eventually try, and I encountered the same problem you have or soon will: No one would talk to me. Especially now, with HIPPA regulations in place, mental health professionals are more and more often saying things like, "I can't even confirm that your brother is a patient of mine, much less talk to you!" It's enough to make you want to scream. And yet, this obstacle is not coming from an evil place, nor is it unmovable.

If you are a family member, remind the therapist
that you can share your observations and concern
without violating confidentiality laws.

If you are a family member, you can share your observations without violating the doctor-patient relationship. If someone tells you he or she can't talk with you, say "I know you can't, and that's not what I am asking you to do. I am not even asking you to verify that my loved one is your patient. All I am asking is that you let me share some observations and concerns about my loved one. All I ask is that you listen for a minute." There are no regulations prohibiting a therapist from listening! Try it and you will see that it opens at least half the line of communication. The other half, getting the therapist to talk with you, requires that you do something further.

As I mentioned earlier, therapists can pave the way for this type of collaboration by clarifying the limits of confidentiality with their patient up front. ("I would like to hear from your family from time to time to get a feel for how they think you're doing. Also, if you become sick, I may want to talk with them to get their help."). The bottom line is that if the patient knows that certain types of communication will occur between doctor and family, confidentiality is not being violated. The rules have to be a little different when you are dealing with serious mental illnesses because judgment and insight can become severely impaired. That's why we all need to talk to one another and work as a team.

When families work actively with the treatment team, they increase the quality of care. It's not something we're proud of, but most doctors and therapists will feel more accountable when a family member is actively involved. Better yet, we become much better at detecting and responding to any worsening of the illness than when we work in isolation.

When I give talks, I often discuss the vital importance of building a "Treatment Triad." What I mean by this is building teamwork among the patient, his loved one, and the mental health professional. When all three are working together, stabilization and/or recovery become much more likely. To become more effective at building a treatment team, you must overcome some common barriers, including the ones I mentioned above. Also, you must identify personal barriers such as your own negative preconceptions about "the other side."

If you're a therapist, you have to overcome your preconceived belief that family members may distract you from your work. One misconception I have had is that family members call me to vent and get free therapy. I am not proud of that thought, but I often have it when I am ending a very long day and a family member wants to talk to me about how hard their relative's illness has been on them.

Of course I understand and sympathize but that's not the point. The problem is, if you have more than one patient (which we all do), that it's impossible to be available to all your patients' involved family members in this way. What I have learned, however, is that if I explain my limitations and suggest that the stressed relative think about getting help for him- or herself, it helps to refocus the conversation on what we should be talking about. If the family member is unwilling to get professional help, I will strongly suggest he or she go to a NAMI meeting to gain support from other people in similar situations.

Don't call to vent. Call a friend, relative, or your own therapist to get that kind of support.

If you're a family member, you may make the mistake of thinking that an unresponsive therapist (one who won't return phone calls, won't talk to you, etc.) doesn't care. I can't tell you that you would be wrong, but I can say that in my experience this assumption is, more likely than not, incorrect. Most therapists (RNs, MSWs, PhDs, PsyDs, and yes, even MDs) got into this line of work because they care. They chose the career because, like me, it has personal meaning for them and they want to help. But if that's the case, why do they sometimes appear so uncaring?

In short, the reason is often "burnout." That said, however, you can help by being focused on specific issues when you call. ("I want to tell you about some warning signs of relapse I'm seeing," or "I'm concerned about the discharge plan because..." Don't call to vent. Call a friend, relative, or your own therapist to get that kind of support.

Finding and Using a Mobile Crisis Team

While maintaining contact and working with doctors is the best possible solution, doing that is not always possible. If you are dealing with a loved one who is an adult, who has never been committed, and who refuses to see a doctor, you may find that you have no one to call. Even if this is the situation, however, you needn't feel that you are alone or have only the police as a resource. That was, in fact, my situation when Henry was committed for the first time. What I didn't take advantage of, however, is the fact that most hospitals with a psychiatric care unit also have a mobile crisis team. This team is usually made up of master's level psychologists, social workers, or nurses who perform home visits. Like paramedics, they're typically in close contact with a doctor who is stationed in the psychiatric emergency room. Mobile crisis teams are trained to evaluate, refer to outpatient treatment, and, if necessary, hospitalize. To find out whether your community has a mobile crisis team, you should call your local hospital and ask for the psychiatric emergency room. Usually, a psychiatric nurse will answer your call, or, if not, the psychiatrist on call. Explain that you are concerned about a loved one and ask what resources are available. The nurse or doctor will be able to tell you about the mobile crisis team and how to contact them. Add this number to your list of doctors and emergency numbers. Sometimes just knowing that it is there can be a relief.

You will also be able to ask about other outpatient services in your community. Even if you haven't reached a crisis point with your loved one, you should feel free to call the psychiatric emergency room or any other local mental health facility. Don't worry about interrupting someone in the middle of an emergency. If you have, he or she will let you know and ask you to call back. When I was covering the psychiatric emergency room during my training, I spent as much time fielding such calls as I did evaluating patients in the ER.

Calling 911 and Asking for CIT Officers

If you call 911, be sure to ask if the law enforcement department you have reached (metro police, sheriff's department, highway patrol, etc.) has a Crisis Intervention Team (CIT). Many now do and many more will have them by the time this book hits the presses. Ask specifically for a CIT-trained unit to respond.

CIT officers have been trained in how to separate criminal behavior from mental illness and, more importantly, how to communicate effectively with an agitated person suffering from psychosis. At LEAP Institute, we have provided adjunctive training seminars for CIT officers around the country. In my experience, those officers who volunteer for the extra training — as much as 40 hours of additional classroom time involving reading, lectures and role-plays — are compassionate and understanding, and have the skills to help calm someone who is psychotic and paranoid or simply frightened. They arrive at the scene with safety first and foremost on their minds but also with the awareness that they are dealing with a person who has mental illness and who needs to be listened to, calmed down and convinced to come safely and quietly for an evaluation.

The Evaluation

After you take your loved one to the hospital or call the mobile crisis team or CIT officers, you should immediately ask to speak with the doctor who conducted or supervised the evaluation. There are several reasons why it is important for you to speak with the doctor in charge of your loved one's case sooner rather than later. The first is the obvious reason discussed above: You are forming a team with the doctors to ensure that your loved one gets the care that he needs. There is currently no cure for serious mental illnesses, so it's a good idea to build a network of people who will be familiar with you and your loved one.

Another reason to make sure you talk with the doctor in charge may sound a bit cynical, but it is not. It is realistic. Sometimes doctors working in hospitals don't have the time or resources to give everyone the quality of attention that may be warranted. If you are a mental health professional, it is usually easier to get the doctor's attention. If you are a family member, you may be asked to call back in the morning. In either case, don't be put off. Act as you would if you were dealing with an accident or the flare-up of some other medical illness like heart disease. In these instances, you would no doubt approach the doctor to find out all the details of the diagnosis, prognosis, and treatment. Find out what's going on and what the plan is. If nothing else is gained, you will at least have let the doctor know that his patient is your loved one and that you hold him accountable for the care that is given.

The doctor who does the diagnosis and intake for your loved one is going to be your biggest ally if your loved one needs to stay in the hospital longer than the 72 hours generally mandated by an emergency commitment. The three-day holding period is all that many states allow without some kind of civil court hearing. (The admitting doctor will be experienced with the commitment procedure for your state.) The length of stay ordered will depend, in large part, on the recommendations of the doctors caring for your loved one.

One Final Word about Calling the Police

The idea of having to call the police for help with a loved one seems very dramatic and somehow wrong. After all, we usually call the police when a crime has been committed. However, you may need to call the police when your loved one is out of control because they're trained to act in situations where people are not in control of their behavior.

Even so, not all police departments offer CIT training. If your local police department doesn't, contact the Memphis, Tennessee Police Department to learn of their crisis intervention program or check with the websites I gave you above. The Memphis PD's CIT program was recognized at a White House conference in 1999 as a model system for "decriminalizing" the mentally ill. Ask for literature and pass it along to your local police.

I was fortunate, in that when I called the Tucson police about my brother in the early 1980s, they had received such specialized training. Nevertheless, whenever I called the police to ask for help getting my brother to the hospital, my mother would become angry with me. She felt protective of Henry and believed that involving the police was somehow criminalizing him.

If you had a five-year-old child who ran into the street, you would pick him up and restrain him. If he had a temper tantrum and threatened to harm you, you would send him to his room.

One explanation I gave my mother then and have since given many family members and mental health professionals is the following: If you had a five-year-old child who ran into the street, you would pick him up and restrain him. If he had a temper tantrum and threatened to harm you, you would probably send him to his room. When someone is a full-grown adult, you can't physically do any of these things. But the police can.

In my experience, police officers usually restrain and transport people with mental illness with respect and dignity.

In my experience, police officers usually restrain and transport mentally ill people with respect and dignity. If you feel that your local police force has not received the training they need to elevate their understanding and sensitivity to persons with serious mental illness, contact your police chief, sheriff, or police commissioner and suggest that they learn about the model used by the Memphis police department (see www.NAMI.org for information).

Very often when you call the police, there will be a scene — your loved one will resist being taken to the hospital. But that isn't always the case—sometimes the police come and are not able to help because everything looks fairly normal and calm. I used to work on a mobile crisis team, and we would call this sudden calmness the "ambulance cure."

We coined the phrase after evaluating a man with schizophrenia who had been screaming threats at the top of his lungs in a 24-hour convenience store. He accused the clerks of spying on him and demanded that they stop. He was delusional and hearing voices that he told us about when we arrived.

After conferring with the psychiatrist at the hospital on our radios, we all agreed that he should be brought in for a 72-hour observation period. However, by the time the ambulance arrived to transport him to the hospital, he was visibly calmer. And by the time he was being evaluated by the ER psychiatrist, he was denying that any of it had happened. He knew that if he talked about the voices or his paranoid fears the doctor would admit him to the hospital. And since he didn't think he was ill, and didn't want to stay, he avoided the topics he knew would get him admitted.

Fortunately, the psychiatrists we worked with trusted our judgment and did not make rash decisions, and after three hours in the ER, he began to get agitated again. He started mumbling to his voices and talking about his concern that the clerks had bugged the interview room.

If your loved one has calmed down by the time the police arrive, be sure to tell them, in detail, everything that happened. If threats were made, don't be shy about talking about them. If furniture was turned over and dishes broken, don't straighten up prior to their arrival. Be certain to tell them that they're dealing with someone who has a history of serious mental illness and that you are very concerned for his safety. Ask them to take your loved one to the hospital if they don't offer to do so. If they refuse, ask to speak with their supervisor.

Below are some tips to help you when you call the police:

- Always ask first for a CIT officer (remembering that the department you reach may not have such a program yet).
- Remember that police officers are often, but not always, trained to deal with someone who is mentally ill.
- Make it clear to the dispatcher that the situation involves someone who is mentally ill. That way the police will be aware of what they're walking into.
- If possible, meet the police at the door, tell them where your loved one is, why you are concerned, and what kind of behavior they will encounter when they enter.
- Be sure to tell them whether or not your loved one has access to any type of weapon. If there is no weapon, the officers will be less anxious and can focus first on the safety of your loved one. If there is a weapon, they need to know.
- If your loved one has thrown or broken anything, don't try to clean up before the police come. Whatever damage your loved has caused may be the only overt sign of illness the officers can see.

Finally, if you need to call the police to help you with your loved one, please don't blame yourself for doing something awful or inappropriate. The police regularly respond to situations involving people who are seriously mentally ill. Also, remember that you are not alone. The Resources section at the back of this book lists organizations that help families who are dealing with mental illness, and many of the websites offer personal accounts of how other people have handled the same or similar situations.

14

How to Survive an Involuntary Treatment

Even if you believe that seeking an involuntary commitment was the best thing for your loved one, you will probably suffer some emotional fallout. You know that your loved one is sick and you know that, at least for the time being, forcing him to take medication was imperative and maybe the only chance he will ever have to get better.

But, he is likely to feel betrayed by what you have done and to not be very open to talking with you about why you did what you did. Worse yet, you may feel that he is right. If either of you believes you have acted like a Judas, there can be no partnership or treatment agreement. That is one of the reasons that dealing with his feelings of betrayal is vital. The other reason, of course, is to regain trust and preserve your relationship.

During the initial days your loved one is in the hospital, it is only natural that he will be angry with you. Wouldn't you be angry if you thought you were not ill and someone had called the police on you, resulting in your being forced into a psychiatric ward? I would be furious! Add to the anger the fact that your loved one is probably sicker than usual (otherwise, why do what you did?) and it may not be possible for you to have a meaningful conversation just yet.

It is imperative that you visit as often as you can
without overburdening yourself.

This doesn't mean that you should avoid going to the hospital to visit. Sometimes well-meaning hospital staff may encourage you to wait if they feel you will be upset to see your loved one so ill; other times, your loved one may refuse to see you. Nevertheless, it is imperative that you visit as often as you can without overburdening yourself. The reason for this is that many people who are forced into the hospital feel that their families want to get rid of them and have abandoned them. It's harder for them to believe this if you try to visit the hospital every day, or close to that, even if it's only for five minutes to say, "Hi, I love you." And if you cannot visit for some reason (e.g., during the COVID-19 epidemic), then make regular phone calls.

During Henry's first real hospitalization, after the time he had been turned away at the ER, he refused to speak with me when I visited. I remember the first time I walked in. He was sitting in front of the television in the common room (called the "day room" in most hospitals). When I went over to him and said hi, he gave me one quick angry look, got up, and went directly to his room. I asked the nurse to get him, but she reported that he didn't want to talk with me and suggested I leave.

Over the next two weeks, I went back again and again despite the fact that I mostly sat in the day room and read the newspaper. It was a long drive to the hospital, so I figured I might as well make the most of my effort and stay a while. More than that, however, I also felt very guilty about what had happened and hoped that if I stayed long enough Henry might come out of his room and agree to talk with me.

Eventually, he did, and at the time I had the good sense to apologize. Although, as I've said, I did some stupid things as well, that apology was a vital first step toward repairing the damage done to our relationship by his hospitalization.

When I encourage you to visit or call, however, I'm basing my recommendation not only on my experience as a family member but also on my experience as a doctor who has worked in several wards like the one my brother was in. I see how patients react when family does not visit. I see how easy it is to feed the seeds of feeling betrayed and how that affects what happens after discharge from the hospital.

So, do your best to visit or call regularly, but, at the same time, remember to take care of yourself during this period. If trips to the hospital are draining and too overwhelming, stay just for the few minutes it takes for your loved one to see that you are there and haven't abandoned him. Then go home and try to relax, watch a movie, go out to dinner with a close friend.

It is important that you talk about what you did and about how it made your loved one feel.

Brooding endlessly about what's going on in the hospital will not help anyone and can be detrimental to you and your relationship with your loved one. If you are not seeing a therapist of your own, this may be a good opportunity for you to find someone you can talk to about your situation. Family organizations like NAMI are particularly helpful in this regard.

At some point during or after the hospitalization, you will need to begin looking for an opportunity to talk with your loved one about what happened. It is important that you talk about what you did and about how it made your loved one feel. There is no perfect script for what you should say in this conversation other than making certain that you are speaking from your heart and touching on the themes I describe below. It may be as simple as when I said to my brother, "I had to call the police. I couldn't have lived with myself if I hadn't." Or, "I know you feel angry and betrayed, but I would have felt guilty and as if I had let you down if I hadn't gotten you into the hospital."

Turning Betrayal into Loyalty

A conversation aimed at dealing with feelings of betrayal should always start with an apology and the statement that you understand how your loved one feels. "I know you don't feel you needed this and I know you are angry with me. I'm very sorry that what I've done is so hurtful to you, but I would like to tell you why I felt I had to do it." In large part, this conversation is more of an apology than a justification, and you need to be careful not to become accusatory or defensive in any way. Acknowledge your loved one's feelings of betrayal while pointing out that you were following your conscience.

I am not recommending that you apologize for what you did,
but rather for how it made your loved one feel.

You may balk at the notion of apologizing. After all, you were acting in your loved one's best interest so you have nothing to be sorry for. I agree. I am not recommending that you apologize for what you did, but rather for how it made your loved one feel. You and I would feel the same way and appreciate the empathy that is conveyed with an apology.

Here are some general do's and don'ts to help you to have a conversation that will aid in mending the relationship.

Do
1. Acknowledge his feelings of betrayal.
2. Ask for forgiveness.
3. Explain why you felt you had to do what you did.
4. Be honest that you would do it again.

Don't
1. Deny his feelings of betrayal.
2. Expect to be forgiven right away.
3. Blame your loved one for what you felt you had to do.
4. Be misleading about what you would do in the future.

There are four main points you should try to convey to your loved one: your regret, your fear that he will be angry with you and not understand your perspective, why you felt you had to take the actions that you did, and an appeal for his forgiveness.

1. Regret
It is very natural that you may feel regret about "locking up" your loved one. It's not unlike the regret we feel whenever we impose a restriction on a child (e.g., when you tell a child "go to your room"). The fact that it was done with the best of intentions doesn't mean that it was easy to do or that you are not sorry you felt you had to do it.

When you have the conversation with your loved one, let him know that you regret having had to commit him and wish you didn't feel you had to do it. But don't blame your loved one for putting you in the position of having to do something you'd rather not have done; this will only lead to estrangement, not an alliance. Instead, simply state your feelings. You feel sorry that your conscience led you to do something you know your loved one felt was hurtful. In the space below, write down any feelings of regret you have about the commitment and how you might say this to your loved one.

Did you write something you will be able to convey to your loved one in a way that helps him understand the dilemma you were in? Put yourself in the shoes of your loved one for a moment and read what you wrote. Is it something you would respond to well? Would you feel blamed? Or do you feel that you would understand how the person who committed you felt about doing it?

Emphasize that your values and love led you to do what you did, not that you were "right" to do it.

Don't speak in absolute truths like, "I had to do this. I had no other choice." Instead say, "I felt I had to do this, I felt I had no other choice." Emphasize that your values and love led you to do what you did, not that you were "right" to do it.

After I learned to talk to my brother in this way, I would say, "I wish I didn't feel the way I do, I am so sorry that I pushed this on you. I know you don't agree with my view, but I hope you can forgive me. I only did this because I felt it was the right thing and because I love you." From there, the conversation generally went something like this.

"If you loved me, you would never have called the police on me. I am angry!"

"Henry, I would feel the same way."

"Then why did you do it?"

"Because—and I wish I didn't feel this way because I know it's hurtful to you—but because I was scared and felt you needed to be in the hospital."

"You've been brainwashed by the psychiatrists. There's nothing wrong with me."

"I understand and respect your perspective. Do you get mine?"

"You were scared and thought you were trying to help me."

"Right. And I am really sorry we're so far apart on this but glad you can at least understand that however misguided I am, my intentions were good. Do you believe that?"

"I do," he said, much to my relief.

By empathizing and normalizing his experience of what I had done to him (saying "I would feel the same way"), I opened the door to Henry's being able to see the important truth, which is, that regardless of who was right (him or me) about his being sick, I did what I did because I felt it was the right thing to do and because I loved him.

2. Fears

Explain what it is you were afraid would happen if you didn't have your loved one committed. Preface your fears by acknowledging that your loved one did not share your concern. ("I know you weren't worried about...") Then ask if he would like to hear what you were worried about. ("Can I tell you why I was worried?")

As you explain the fears you had, it is important that you phrase them in such a way that you are not making accusations about anticipated behavior. Also, explain that your fears grew out of the fact that you care for him so deeply — not from expecting him to behave badly. Keeping in mind what was said above, write down a few of the fears you think you could share with your loved one to help him understand your motivations and mend the relationship.

Have a look at what you wrote and refer to the do's and don'ts given above. Did you follow the advice I gave? How would you feel if the tables were turned and you were hearing your words played back to you? If you think you would feel cared for and not defensive, you are on the right track.

Don't ask him to agree — ask only that he understand and forgive you for following your conscience.

3. Actions

Explain why you took the actions you did. Remind your loved one of the event(s) that precipitated your calling the police (or crisis team) or taking him to the hospital. In my case with Henry, it was his expressing suicidal thoughts and my fear that he would harm himself. As you write down the reasons for your actions, keep in mind that you don't want to sound accusing or angry. This is a conversation in which you are trying to convey your reasons for having your loved one committed. Don't ask him to agree — ask only that he understand and forgive you for following your conscience. In the space provided, write down the reasons you pursued a commitment.

By now, you know what I am going to ask. Have a look at what you wrote and see if you followed the do's and don'ts given above. Next, ask yourself how you would feel if the tables were turned and you were hearing your words played back to you. Would you feel like arguing against the points made or would you be able to hear them without getting defensive?

4. Appeal for forgiveness and understanding

What you are asking your loved one to do is try to comprehend why you did what you had to do, how much you love him, and how much his forgiveness means to you. Don't be afraid to let him have the upper hand. In other words, stand firmly on your convictions but don't try to justify yourself or your decision. After all, you won! Think of the power you wielded. Your loved one was forced to take medicine or forced into a hospital against his will. (How can he be forced to take medicine without being forced into the hospital?) You can afford to be magnanimous. You are asking your loved one to forgive you; that is all. Listen carefully to what he has to say and see where the dialogue leads.

If your loved one refuses to talk with you about the commitment, write it all down in a letter or text.

Don't expect to be successful after only one conversation. It will take several discussions before your loved one's misconceptions about how you feel and why you did what you did can be corrected. If your loved one refuses to talk with you about the commitment, write it all down in a letter or text message. In fact, even if you have had successful discussions, it's useful to write a letter or text that covers the four points discussed above. Serious mental illness sometimes makes it difficult for people to remember. Having your explanation and appeal for forgiveness in writing will help your loved one remember what you said.

I wish I could end this chapter by saying that if you follow all the above steps you will have turned your loved one's feelings of betrayal into feelings of understanding and empathy for your predicament. But that would be unrealistic. Whether your loved one is able to forgive, let go of feeling betrayed, and understand your point of view will rely in large part on his innate capacity to accomplish these things. However, I can promise that if you follow the advice given here, you will feel better about what you have done and reduce the degree of conflict in your relationship with your loved one.

15

The Surprise

I'm sure you remember that one of the first things I told you, way back at the beginning of this book, was that your goal was not to get your loved one to admit he or she was sick but to get him to follow his statement "I'm not sick" with the statement "But, I could use some help." In other words, the techniques I've been teaching you are not aimed at getting the person who is mentally ill to gain insight into being ill; they are directed specifically at getting him to find reasons to accept treatment despite what he believes.

If you've reached the point where your patient or loved one has made that commitment, what you want to do now is make sure you don't revert to old bad habits like giving your opinion without first asking if the other person wants to hear it. You need to maintain and build on the collaborative dialogue you've begun, and while you may be tempted to remind the mentally ill person that "doctor knows best," or even worse, "father knows best," you've got to remember that those so-called wise words aren't going to make one bit of difference to the one you're trying to help. In fact, they will more than likely just blow up the bridge you've so carefully been building between you.

But you know all that already, right? So what's the surprise? The surprise is that when people with a serious mental illness are in treatment and when they have the kind of relationship I've been trying to help you build with them—one that allows them to feel their point of view is respected and to trust you—they may begin to develop insight.

Remember Vicky, whose interview with Dr. Kohut you read in Chapter 6? Initially, Vicky continued to believe she was "cured" of bipolar disorder but agreed to continue taking her lithium on a trial basis for six months and then, if she decided to go off it, to do so in conjunction with her doctor. She was able to make this commitment because Dr. Kohut had allowed her to understand that she was, ultimately, the one in charge of whether or not she would take the medicine—by doing that, he won her trust and showed her that he honored and respected her feelings. After a while, Vicky was also able to see what happened when she lowered her dose or discontinued her medication, and she gained true insight into the relationship between taking the medication and remaining asymptomatic. When she recognized that without the lithium she was getting "worn out" again, she asked to be put back on medication.

And then there was Dolores, who kept losing jobs because she was holding conversations aloud with the voices in her head. At first, Dolores didn't see any relationship between her getting fired and going off her medication. In fact, she initially believed that the medication was making her hear voices. It took a long time, and several more hospitalizations, but Dolores did gradually come to have some insight into the fact that when she stopped taking medication she talked to herself more, and that this was likely to make people think she was "nuts." Like Vicky, she developed insight into how medications helped her with a problem she was having. Vicky didn't call the problem "bipolar disorder"; she called it getting "worn out." Dolores's problem, as she saw it, wasn't having hallucinations; it was talking aloud to herself. Nevertheless, both of these women developed insight into how the medications helped them with their problems as they saw them. The surprise, then, is that over time people do begin to redefine their problems as mental illness, whether or not they define mental illness in exactly the same way you do.

In psychology, we call this the "change paradox." When you stop pushing someone to change, often they find reasons to change all on their own. I think that is what happened not only with Vicky and Dolores but also with other patients who have benefited from the kind of relationship I've been talking about while taking their medications. Given the room to explore their situation with someone they trusted and who did not preach or tell them they were sick, they were able to develop insight. First the insight was about positive outcomes linked to taking medicine and then later, into having a mental illness.

We know today, right now, that building a respectful and trusting relationship is the key to helping someone with poor insight accept treatment for mental illness.

I think the anecdotal evidence is pretty compelling, but there are also scientific studies to show that developing the kinds of relationships I've been talking about can and does ameliorate lack of insight in patients with serious mental illness. In a study by Dr. Roisen Kemp and her colleagues, published in the British Journal of Psychiatry in 1998, the researchers found that medication adherence and insight improved over an 18-month follow-up period after only six sessions of MET. (LEAP is partially based on MET, which seeks to create a collaborative relationship with the person in "denial.") This is one good example of how building the mutually respectful and trusting relationships we have been talking about can help with both adherence and insight. And, as I mentioned in Chapter 10, new research on medication may also help in our battle against anosognosia. Regardless of what happens with the research on medication, however, we know today—right now—that building a respectful and trusting relationship is the key to helping someone with poor insight accept treatment.

Whether you are a family member or a mental health provider, what this means is that when you create a non-judgmental and trusting relationship, the person you are trying to help will find reasons to be in treatment. It may take a year or two of staying in treatment, but the pay-off over a lifetime is incalculable.

As you go forward, however, you need to remember that you are a member of the team. You need to be strong and well rested. If you do more than you should, you will lose motivation and risk "burnout." Burnout is a term used by mental health professionals to describe the feeling of complete exhaustion that comes from having been immersed in other people's problems for too long. Exhausting yourself will only make you less effective and your loved one or patient feel like a burden.

If you are a family member, I want to add one final word from one family member to another. You are in a unique position to help your loved one learn how to cope with mental illness. You knew your loved one before the illness struck, which means that you also know the core person who is often eclipsed by symptoms of the disease. When someone who is seriously mentally ill feels that you see him for who he is, and not just for the diagnosis he has been given, he will be open to learning from you.

The Surprise for Henry and Xavier

Henry never developed insight into being mentally ill. But the last time I saw him, in the days following our mother's funeral, I can't tell you how much comfort I received from him—it was more visceral than verbal. I know he felt the same. Yes, we talked, but our shared battles, betrayals and ultimately our reconciliation, made possible by our respect for each other, was something we felt in our bones.

On the drive back to his house, on our last night together, my brother told me he felt I saw him for who he was. Henry was very kind, smart, funny, insightful (about most things), and creative. Yes, he was a pain in the ass (and I to him) during the early years of his illness when we argued about whether or not he was mentally ill and needed treatment. But I was to blame for that more than he. Henry was able to laugh at life. I saw him and liked him and he knew that.

I learned a lot from my brother—a man most people gave a wide berth to because of his explosive eruptions into laughter for no apparent reason and his conversations with the voices only he heard. He taught me how to throw a baseball, ride a bicycle, and the power of humility. When we were growing up, he brought humor and magic into my life (like the time, when I was five, that he convinced me I had just missed Santa Claus flying by our window). More recently, he taught me about compassion, patience, perseverance and most importantly, forgiveness. I feel very fortunate, as you will read in the next section, that we had a strong friendship for many years before he died.

LEAP would not exist if not for Henry Amador. It was not my creation alone or that of my collaboration with Aaron (Tim) Beck, M.D. and other colleagues and patients. More than anyone else, Henry helped me to develop LEAP and without it, I am sure we would have lost many years of closeness, laughter and love.

In the next, and last, section of this book I give you the details of where LEAP comes from theoretically, a summary of recent research on cognitive behavioral therapy for schizophrenia (which LEAP draws on in part) and a review of recent research on the link between violence and poor adherence. I next make an argument for why we must include anosognosia in our diagnostic manual, not only for schizophrenia, but for other psychotic disorders.

Finally, I tell you the end of Henry's story. Perhaps "end" is not the correct word because I believe that with every copy of this book that is read, his story will continue to unfold — and his compassion, empathy and kindness will help others reach people with serious mental illness and bring them back to their families.

Part IV

Theory, Research and Practical Advice on LEAP

16

LEAP Theory and Research

The first edition of this book described LEAP in 2000. However, LEAP draws from pre-existing psychotherapeutic traditions that date back 60 years. LEAP has three major influences: Carl Rogers's "Client-Centered Therapy," Aaron T. Beck's "Cognitive Therapy," and Miller and Rollnick's "Motivational Interviewing."

Carl Rogers's Client-Centered Therapy (1951, 1959)

LEAP is partly based on Rogers's conception of the transformative power of "actively listening" to patients:

> *"Real communication occurs...when we listen with understanding. What does this mean? It means to see the expressed idea and attitude from the other person's point of view, to sense how it feels to him, to achieve his frame of reference in regard to the thing he is talking about."* (Carl Rogers, 1961; *On Becoming a Person*, Mariner Books, page 332)

The main idea is that judgment or evaluation is a barrier to constructive communication. The better you listen, the less you judge. When the patient feels understood, he feels trust and openness to the therapist.

Among the main lessons I learned from Client-Centered Therapy was that I should give up the directive-expert perspective, communicate respect for the client's views, listen actively and show empathy.

Aaron Beck's Cognitive Therapy (1979)

In 1979, Aaron T. Beck, in his book Cognitive Therapy of Depression, highlights that specific dysfunctional cognitive patterns lead to or sustain mental disorders. However, to listen is not enough in order to modify these specific dysfunctional cognitive patterns (called schema). Cognitive therapy offers many techniques that are helpful to improve a patient's engagement into the interaction and ultimately treatment. Thus, when working on the issue of adherence to treatment, the therapist should:

- Take a collaborative stance.
- Use mutually agreed on agendas.
- Explore disadvantages and advantages of medication and services.
- Define goals that the patient is willing to work on.

Among the many lessons I learned from Cognitive Therapy was the importance of creating structure when possible, such as beginning meetings with setting an agenda — but staying flexible.

Attempt to create an agenda for conversations either by following the patient's lead (e.g., "You were just talking about how angry you are that the police picked you up. Can we talk about that today?") or introducing ideas (e.g., "You mentioned not liking medication. Can we talk about that?").

Remember to ask questions. Cognitive therapy is very collaborative, as is LEAP, and the therapist frequently "checks in" with the patient to find out what is perceived as helpful and what is not. Importantly, cognitive therapy also relies on conducting cost/benefit analyses with the client—just as we do in LEAP—whenever possible.

Motivational Interviewing (1991)

"Motivational Interviewing, or Motivational Enhancement Therapy (MET) is an approach to helping people change that was originally developed by William R. Miller and Stephen Rollnick. It directly addresses a significant problem common to all therapies: resistance to change. In MET, resistance is seen as a result of ambivalence about change. Its primary goals are to help clients increase their intrinsic motivation and resolve ambivalence in order to facilitate behavior change." Hal Arkowitz et al., (2008) Motivational Interviewing in the treatment of psychological problems, London: The Guilford Press, Page ix.

In Motivational Interviewing, the therapist is a guide who asks questions, listens and ultimately informs his patients. As you will see, LEAP was influenced mainly by these first two components of Motivational Interviewing.

Like in MI, LEAP's main focus is to obtain collaboration from the patient by showing respect for his autonomy and opinions even when they are at odds with the therapist's. However, LEAP differs from MET in its approach to informing (i.e., giving an opinion, making recommendations or educating).

The main idea is that the therapist should adopt a guiding style (e.g., use open-ended questions) rather than a controlling or directive one in order to promote a more active involvement in the interaction. Consequently, the therapist strives to:

- Guide rather than press (using open-ended questions).
- Assess motivation for change.
- Support the client's self-efficacy.
- Assess previous attempts to fix the problem.
- Talk in hypothetical language for patients who are less ready to change.

- Collaboratively explore ambivalence to motivate the process of behavior change.

Among the lessons learned from MET is to not direct. LEAP takes this a big step further in that we encourage you to show genuine reluctance to direct—to give your opinion. Like MET, LEAP also capitalizes on those aspects of insight the person has and ignores those that appear deeply ingrained (such as the belief "I am not sick"). Instead, we focus on the desire to change certain things in the person's life, to articulate and strive for goals and to resolve ambivalence about getting help to achieve those goals.

Summary

In Carl Rogers's Client-Centered Therapy, as well as in Motivational Interviewing, the process of building an alliance starts by focusing on understanding the patient's perspectives and problems. Understanding the patient's perspective is central to the LEAP approach. Understanding and communicating that perspective accurately is considered the key to transforming an adversarial relationship into an alliance.

As opposed to Rogers's Client Centered Therapy, as well as Beck's Cognitive Therapy, however, MET focuses on listening to and working on ambivalence and "change talk." Change talk is based on the patient's desires, ability, reasons and need for change:

- What the patient *desires* ("What do you want?")
- The patient's *ability* ("What can you do?")
- The *reasons* for change ("Why would you do it? Why would you change?")
- The *need* for change ("How much do you need to change?")

In short, LEAP utilizes the following tools and principles from the three therapies:

From Rogers's Client-Centered Therapy: Reflective listening as the foundation for creating an alliance. Central to this technique is a complete lack of judgment—no opinion about what is being said is given unless it has been asked for (preferably many times over).

From Cognitive Therapy: The collaborative stance, setting an agenda and cost benefit analyses.

From MI: The patient remains the final arbiter of the change process. Ambivalence about change is explored. And perhaps most importantly, internal and external motivators (or desires) are identified.

I admit it. LEAP is not entirely new. Its main principles are familiar, so sometimes people will say, "LEAP is just like…" They are not so much accusing me of plagiarism as much as recognizing the heritage.

The American folk singer Woody Guthrie, writer of the song "This Land is Your Land," which we all learned as children, was sometimes accused of stealing the melodies for his songs from old gospel tunes. In fact, he had never tried to hide his practice of borrowing from melodies that had already been written, saying, "There are no new melodies; they're all used up!"

I feel that way about most useful insights into human psychology and relations. LEAP is new, but like Guthrie's songs, it relies on what came before—from certain philosophical traditions, from the three therapies I summarized above, and from common sense. It is a method for easily remembering and using age-old truths in your everyday life. Like a melody that is catchy and hard to forget, once you learn LEAP, you will find that you can call it up any time you need it.

Research on LEAP

Next, I briefly describe the results of a study my colleagues Celine Paillot, Ph.D., Raymond Goetz, Ph.D., and I published in the National Institute of Mental Health's Journal *Schizophrenia Bulletin*. The study was presented at the International Congress on Schizophrenia Research in June of 2009. Although Dr. Goetz and I consulted with her and published the study together, Dr. Paillot conducted the study herself while pursuing her doctorate degree at the University of Paris.

As stated earlier, most patients with *DSM-IV*-diagnosed schizophrenia exhibited full or partial non-adherence to pharmacological treatment (Rummel-Kluge, 2008). Only about one-third reliably took antipsychotic medication as prescribed (Oehl, 2000). Poor adherence (i.e., both complete and partial non-adherence) was found to be associated with relapse, increased involuntary admissions, poorer course of illness, and increased incidence of violence and suicide (Amador and David, 2004). Given the serious outcomes associated with poor adherence, interventions aimed at improving and maintaining adherence were of great interest to clinicians, researchers, and policy-makers.

The main aim of our study was to assess the efficacy of LEAP when compared to a control intervention. The study involved 54 patients diagnosed with schizophrenia about to be discharged following inpatient treatment. Patients were randomly assigned to either the experimental or control therapies. Subjects did not know whether they were receiving the experimental versus control therapy which was essentially Carl Rogers's Client-Centered Therapy as described above.

All patients were treated with long-acting injectable antipsychotic medications (either typical or atypical) and rated as compliant when the injection was confirmed and noncompliant if the injection was refused or the appointment for the injection was missed. Insight into schizophrenia and attitudes toward treatment were assessed using the Scale to Assess Unawareness of Mental Disorder, the Birchwood Insight Scale and the Drug Attitude Inventory, respectively. All assessments were made by a single rater who was blind to group assignment.

The results show that compared to Rogers's therapy, LEAP improved motivation for change, insight and adherence to treatment. This study found LEAP to be superior to the control psychotherapy. It improved compliance, motivation for change, insight and attitudes towards treatment.

Among the strengths of the experimental design was the fact that we used randomized blinded group assignment, blinded assessments of the dependent variables and near 100% reliability and validity of the adherence measure. Among the limitations of the study was the absence of a LEAP fidelity measure and the fact that the senior author (Dr. Paillot) was the only therapist for all patients. As such, she could have inadvertently biased the results by differentially treating patients depending on which therapy they were assigned to. We are currently planning to attempt a replication of this study in a larger, more heterogeneous sample with a longitudinal assessment of fidelity to the LEAP intervention and therapists blinded to study hypotheses.

17

Psychotherapy for Psychosis?

As I wrote in Chapter 1, and previously in a column for *Schizophrenia Magazine*,[1] about 50% of persons with schizophrenia have great difficulty seeing that they have a mental illness (i.e., they have the symptom of anosognosia) and this lack of awareness is linked to frontal lobe dysfunction. As such, it does not change—insight does not increase—easily over time.

The data supporting this statement are so well replicated that, as I mentioned before, *DSM 5*, the diagnostic manual all North American doctors and mental health professionals use, reports these facts (American Psychiatric Association Press, 2013).

In addition, as I wrote earlier, many persons with schizophrenia and bipolar disorder either refuse, or take only a small portion of the medication prescribed (estimates are from 50 to 75%). And for those persons who understand that they have an illness and take medication, not all respond to the treatment or respond only partially (e.g., the voices are diminished but the delusions persist). So, if many people refuse medication, or take only sub-therapeutic doses, and medication does not always work for those who do take it as prescribed, what can be done?

---

1 Portions of this chapter and some of the chapters to follow appeared, in part, in a column I wrote in the past for *Schizophrenia Magazine*, now published as a newsletter (www.sardaa.org). The publisher has kindly given me permission to reproduce excerpts from this work here.

*So if many people refuse medication, or take only
sub-therapeutic doses... what can be done?*

Though I pose it as a question in the title of this chapter, I have no doubt that, as a field, we need to offer psychotherapy to most, if not all persons with psychosis. In this chapter, I will highlight some of the research on Cognitive Behavioral Therapy (CBT) in psychosis. I will also briefly discuss "Motivational Interviewing" which I consider a "close cousin" of CBT and argue that strong support exists for their effectiveness in increasing adherence to medication, improving some aspects of insight into illness, lowering the severity of some symptoms, and as importantly, encouraging patients to become active consumers engaged in trying to find the treatments and resources that help them best.

Lessons Learned about Using Psychotherapy in Psychosis

The first lesson I learned was in college, in a classroom in 1978—long term intensive psychoanalysis cures schizophrenia and other forms of "psychotic denial." It does not merely reduce the severity of symptoms, it cures the illness itself! Most often the focus of treatment then was to undo the damage done by the "schizophrenogenic mother" whose style of communicating emotion produced schizophrenia.

The second lesson I learned was years later from the doctor who first diagnosed my brother Henry—the only treatment for schizophrenia was antipsychotic medication and "supportive therapy." Supportive therapy, at the time, appeared to consist of individual meetings and group therapy aimed at "reality testing" which, to my brother's ears sounded a lot like people telling him he was wrong to think the things he did and was "crazy."

Why the Change from Psychoanalysis to Drugs and Reality Testing?

A 1984 landmark study conducted by Yale psychiatrist Dr. Tom McGlashan and his colleagues at the Chestnut Lodge, a nationally renowned treatment center for schizophrenia at the time, showed that psychoanalysis by no means cured schizophrenia and, in most instances, offered very little help at all. Then, in the 1990's, with the National Institute of Mental Health's (NIMH) announcement of the "Decade of the Brain" research initiative for schizophrenia (inspired in large part by family members working with the National Alliance on Mental Illness together with clinicians and scientists), the pendulum swung the other way. Psychotherapy was bad and pharmacotherapy, or drugs, was good. Obviously, this is a gross oversimplification, but for many of us, that was the view.

I gladly joined the chorus of well-intentioned family members, doctors and researchers who preached that antipsychotic drugs were the key to stabilization and recovery and that there was little or no room for psychotherapy which promised more harm than good. In retrospect, we threw the baby out with the bath water.

Although I was trained in psychoanalytic psychotherapy and used it with many patients, I saw how antipsychotic medicines were lowering and even eliminating symptoms of schizophrenia in my brother and in others with related psychotic disorders. I gladly joined the chorus of well-intentioned family members, doctors and researchers who preached that antipsychotic drugs were the key to stabilization and recovery and that there was little or no room for psychotherapy, which promised more harm than good. In retrospect, we threw the baby out with the bath water.

Fortunately, a small group of researchers in the United Kingdom came to the attention of Aaron T. Beck, M.D. from the University of Pennsylvania, the father of cognitive therapy (and my collaborator in the development of an earlier version of LEAP). Together, they began a yearly meeting of scientists studying cognitive therapy in patients with schizophrenia and other psychotic disorders. In June of 2009, I attended their 10th anniversary meeting, which was held at the University of Pennsylvania Medical School. One of my colleagues and I had written a review paper some years before, concluding that CBT had many positive applications for persons with schizophrenia and other psychotic disorders, and the conference helped to cement and expand this view. [2]Here are some of the lessons I learned from the conference and the research literature.

The Good Thing about Psychotherapy

First the bad news: The consensus from the conference seemed to be that CBT was not particularly effective in treating negative symptoms. Also, in the USA, it is very rarely offered when compared to its use in the United Kingdom. The good news is that research conducted since our last review of the literature in 2001 indicates that CBT is effective in treating some positive symptoms of schizophrenia and other psychotic disorders (so-called "positive" symptoms include hallucinations, delusions and thought disorder). Hallucinations, in particular, appear to be helped with CBT.

In our review of the literature in 2001, Dr. Anna Seckinger and I found that poor insight and non-adherence to medication were common and problematic areas that present major stumbling blocks in the treatment of patients suffering from schizophrenia and other psychotic disorders, and that CBT and interventions derived from such approaches (like Motivational Interviewing) improve some aspects of insight into illness, increase adherence

---

2 Seckinger, RA, Amador, XF. "Cognitive-behavioral therapy in schizophrenia." *Journal of Psychiatric Practice*, 2001.

to medication, ameliorate the severity of hallucinations and sometimes delusions, and help with other negative consequences of related psychotic disorders. The papers presented at the 10th Anniversary Conference on CBT in Schizophrenia reaffirmed the main findings of our earlier review.

Also, in a study published in the British Journal of Psychiatry, the authors found that compared to a control therapy, CBT was superior at reducing incidents of aggression in patients with a history of aggression and violence and was superior at reducing delusion severity and decreasing risk management. Furthermore, the treatment was acceptable to the majority of individuals; drop-out rates from CBT therapy were much lower.

Finally, a review of twenty years of psychosocial research aimed at improving medication adherence, published in the *American Journal of Psychiatry* in 2002 (see *http://leapinstitute. org/RESEARCH.html* and click on "Review Paper") found that only those programs that included elements of Motivational Interviewing were effective in helping motivate persons with schizophrenia to accept treatment and stick with it.

Why Psychotherapy Is Rarely Offered

Despite all the evidence—and even more data for the effectiveness of CBT for treating other disorders common in schizophrenia and related psychotic disorders like mood and anxiety disorders—the overwhelming majority of persons with schizophrenia and related psychotic disorders in North America have never been offered a course of treatment with CBT or related therapies (e.g., LEAP).

I think this is for two reasons. First, there is no schizophrenigenic mother. Unfortunately, most clinicians still feel guilt for believing or being part of a field that once preached that bad parenting caused schizophrenia. To them I say: "Get over it. None of us meant to do any harm—we were simply ignorant and stuck in a particular theory that had never been tested." Second, schizophrenia and related psychotic disorders are indeed brain disorders.

‖‖‖

Consumers, relatives, mental health professionals and policymakers tend to focus first and foremost on the brain, all the while forgetting where the brain resides — in a human being.

‖‖‖

The research conducted during the "Decade of the Brain" and after revealed that fact unequivocally. Consequently, consumers, relatives, mental health professionals and policymakers now tend to focus first and foremost on the brain, all the while forgetting where the brain resides — in a human being. Meanwhile, we have never had a multibillion dollar industry promoting consumer and professional education about psychotherapy for schizophrenia and related psychotic disorders. But we have had such deep pockets educating us about the benefits of antipsychotic medicines. This is not a criticism — it is a simple incontrovertible truth.

So it is up to us to become educated about psychotherapies that have been studied and shown to be effective, and up to us to see that both private and public funds are directed toward training the professionals needed to deliver these therapies and make them available in our communities.[3] I don't find this task daunting or impossible because I have already seen much progress made since I opened my first book about schizophrenia and since my brother's first episode of illness.

---

3 For more information on CBT for persons with schizophrenia and related psychotic disorders see: *www.BeckInstitute.org.*

18

Violence and Mental Illness

I woke up searching frantically for my glasses on the night stand—knocking over a glass of water before touching the wire rims. Pulling them on, I saw it was 4 a.m. I was in a cold sweat and my heart was pounding. Henry was pacing in the hallway shouting at the voices only he could hear. The thought to talk with him never entered my mind—I had been up late trying to convince him he needed to go back on the medicine, but all I accomplished was to further agitate him. Listening to his side of a heated argument, I imagined him bursting through the door with a knife in his hand. I swung my legs over the bed and walked to the door with my head hung low in shame and weariness, and locked it.

My research and this book are frequently cited by advocates who promote assisted outpatient treatment (see www.psychlaws. org) and by advocates who oppose involuntary treatments on the grounds they would not be needed if adequate outpatient treatments such as LEAP were available. I can see the wisdom in both sides of the debate. That said, until suicide, gross self-neglect, other forms of self-harm and violence stemming from psychotic states can be reliably controlled, involuntary treatments will always be needed. To turn our heads and look the other way would be immoral and criminal—which brings me to the focus of this chapter.

Are people with schizophrenia more apt to commit violent crimes and acts compared to "the chronically normal," as my good friend, the late Dr. Fred Frese (a consumer and psychologist with schizophrenia), would have said? On a more personal note: Should I have been afraid of my brother whom, before he became ill, I trusted more than anyone?

Research on Violence and Schizophrenia

When giving seminars, I often say, "Individuals with schizophrenia and related psychotic disorders are no more violent than the general population," and then go on to cite the research that backs me up. For nearly two decades, this statement has been a mantra for many of us who are advocates for better treatments, services, and laws for persons with schizophrenia. But more recent, well-replicated research indicates the story is not so simple.

For example, in a recent national study of violent behavior in persons with schizophrenia, the authors found that symptoms of losing contact with reality, such as delusions and hallucinations, increased the odds of serious violence by nearly three times the normal rate. Results of the study, which was conducted with patients in real-world community settings as part of the NIMH-funded Clinical Antipsychotic Trials of Intervention Effectiveness (CATIE), are consistent with previous independent studies. Most studies show that when hallucinations and delusions are worsened, the potential for violence increases dramatically.

As a forensic expert who has worked on more than 30 death-penalty cases involving persons with schizophrenia and related disorders that have committed homicides, I can say unequivocally that the anecdotal evidence is overwhelming. The story was the same in nearly every case I worked on.

When hallucinations, thought disorder, and delusions worsened, the defendants became frightened and angry, and, in some cases, coolly planned how they would commit murder. More often than not, we are talking about people who became paranoid and/or grandiose, people who, for example, felt convinced they had to defend themselves from their relatives who had become possessed by evil spirits, or accomplish some other delusion-based imperative such as saving the earth from alien invasion by killing a radio talk show host who was broadcasting the beacon the aliens were using to coordinate their attack.

Impaired Insight Causes Medication Non-Adherence Which Increases the Risk of Violence

Most persons with schizophrenia and other psychotic disorders, including bipolar disorder, benefit from treatment with antipsychotic medication. When we look at the majority—those who do respond to treatment—we find that the most common cause of medication refusal and partial non-adherence is poor insight.

Consequently, if we want to decrease the rate of violence in the population of persons with schizophrenia and other psychotic disorders, we have to break the cycle caused by poor insight: Believing "I am not sick" leads to the conclusion "I don't need medicine," which in turn, leads to a worsening of those symptoms that cause otherwise peace-loving people with no history of aggression or violence to become violent.

The CATIE study found that participants living with families "they felt listened to them 'most of the time' had half the rate of violence compared to those living with families that did not listen to them."

How do we break that cycle?

Part of the answer lies in the same nationwide study that recently emphasized the well-replicated link between a worsening in psychotic symptoms and violence. The CATIE study found that participants living with families "they felt listened to them 'most of the time' had half the rate of violence compared to those living with families that did not listen to them." If we needed only one reason to try the LEAP Reflective Listening Tool, this would be it.

If they had measured it, I believe the CATIE investigators would have found the same result—less violence in persons working with therapists who listened "most of the time" instead of offering unsolicited advice and debating whether or not their clients were ill. The reason I believe this is that our own research and that of others, shows that communication strategies that emphasize active listening skills—whether used by therapists, friends, or family—create trusting relationships that lead people to accept treatment even when they do not believe they are ill.

Twenty-five years ago, when I was wakened from sleep by my brother's ranting at his hallucinations, should I have locked the door? In light of the recent research and the professional experiences I have had since that night, I have to say the answer is yes. Although he was never violent, he was nevertheless exhibiting some of the warning signs (increased hallucinations, agitation, and paranoid delusions).

At that time, before much of the research on which LEAP is based, and that confirming the impact of long-acting injectable medications on adherence was completed, my only reasonable course of action was to call the police whenever he posed a clear danger to himself and refused treatment. But today, when faced with someone who has poor insight into being ill, I often turn first to LEAP and to long-acting injectable medications to help ensure that persons with schizophrenia and related disorders do not experience a worsening of those symptoms that can lead to violence.

Today, when asked, "Are people with schizophrenia more violent?" I now answer, "No, not when they are in treatment and the symptoms are well controlled."

19

DSM-5 and Anosognosia

For the *DSM IV-TR (text revision)*, my co-chair, Michael Flaum, M.D., and I were asked by the American Psychiatric Association (APA) to revise the text to ensure that it was based on scientific consensus rather than on the views of a single expert. (I had worked on the two previous editions as a *Schizophrenia Expert, Columbia University Field Trial Coordinator*, and in a few other roles.)

To accomplish that revision, we brought together experts from around the United States and overseas to read the research and independently review the text we proposed so that it would accurately reflect the scientific evidence available at the time. Once that process was complete, the text was independently reviewed again by experts on the APA Task Force. At that time, our peer-reviewers and the task force agreed that "*a majority of individuals with schizophrenia lacked insight into having a psychotic illness*" and that this problem was "*a manifestation of the illness itself rather than a coping strategy*" (page 304, *DSM-IV-TR*, APA Press, 2000). It was a symptom of the brain disorder rather than denial. It was compared to anosognosia—an unawareness syndrome seen in stroke patients and others with frontal lobe lesions.

The current *Diagnostic and Statistical Manual for Mental Disorders, 5th Edition (DSM-5)*, expands on the discussion of anosognosia that was first described in the *DSM IV-TR*.

I have quoted this passage from the *DSM 5* several times in this 20th Anniversary Edition of *I Am Not Sick, I Don't Need Help!* Please forgive me for seeming redundant. The reason is that even after twenty years, most psychiatrists and other mental health professionals continue to feel certain that what they are dealing with when a patient says "I am not sick" over a period of months, years and decades is denial! They have never read the *DSM* passage or if they have, they have not read the underlying research. They hold on to the belief that the poor insight they see is a symptom of denial rather than a symptom of the disorder itself and/or a brain dysfunction.

I have spoken frequently all over the United States and overseas for the past 20 years. I have asked my audiences if they have heard of anosognosia and whether they believe this "unawareness syndrome" exists in schizophrenia and related disorders (e.g., schizo-affective disorder and other psychotic illnesses).

In the early years, only one or two hands went up in groups of two hundred or more. Today, between one-half to two-thirds of my audiences raise their hands—whether in Australia, New Zealand, France, Belgium, Hawaii, Hungary, Spain or Ohio (and nearly every other U.S. state).

However, many mental health professionals and family members still have trouble believing it. For this reason—because of the continuing gap between science and practice—I will briefly review the research that has convinced me and most other experts on schizophrenia that when a patient with this disorder (who has received a reliable diagnosis) persists for years in saying, "I am not sick, I don't need help," he is giving voice to a symptom of the illness rather than to denial. Before I do that, I will share what the *DSM 5* has to say about "poor insight":

- Unawareness of illness is typically a symptom rather than a coping strategy. It is comparable to the lack of awareness of neurological deficits following brain damage, termed *anosognosia*.

- This symptom is the most common predictor of nonadherence to treatment. It has been found to predict higher relapse rates, increased number of involuntary treatments, poorer psychosocial functioning, aggression, and a poorer course of illness (page 101).

This widely-used authoritative manual now defines "unawareness of illness" as a *symptom* and that this symptom is comparable to *anosognosia*. What is particularly important is the statement that anosognosia in schizophrenia is *the most common predictor of nonadherence to treatment*—the top reason patients either refuse treatment or drop out of treatment once it is started.

Studies Using Neuropsychological Tests

Numerous studies consistently report that low performance on the Wisconsin Card Sorting Test (WCST) is significantly correlated with insight deficits in patients with schizophrenia (e.g. Shad et. al., 2006; see also the relevant review chapter in Amador and David, *Insight and Psychosis*, edited volume, Oxford University Press, 2004). The WCST measures, among other things, executive functions (anterior cortical function, a.k.a. frontal lobe function) such as self-reflection, planning, rule acquisition, abstract thinking, initiating appropriate actions while inhibiting inappropriate actions. Frontal lobe lesions have been found to be a common cause of anosognosia in neurological disorders (see reviews in: Amador et. al., *Schizophrenia Bulletin*, 1991 and in Amador, X. *I Am Not Sick, I Don't Need Help!* (Vida Press, 2007).

Structural Brain Imaging Studies

Although far fewer in number, studies of the neurobiological underpinnings of poor insight in schizophrenia generally find that anosognosia in schizophrenia is correlated with a range of frontal lobe abnormalities (see Alexander and Struss, 2006; see also the relevant review chapter in: Amador and David, *Insight and Psychosis*, edited volume, Oxford University Press, 2004).

Additional structural and functional brain imaging studies and post-mortem brain studies are currently underway and should help to shed light on the pathophysiology of this common symptom of schizophrenia.

How Research Influenced the DSM-5

Psychiatric diagnoses are purely descriptive. To date, there is no blood test or brain scan that can diagnose mental illness. We look instead for diagnostic categories and dimensions that tell us something about what is likely to happen to the person (i.e., we ask, "What is the predictive value or validity of the diagnostic category or subtype?"). This also helps us to choose and recommend treatments and services that will be helpful to the individual.

The previous subtypes of schizophrenia (e.g., catatonic, undifferentiated, disorganized, etc.) have limited predictive value. For that reason—and because the extensive research on poor insight in schizophrenia indicates that patients with this symptom have a poorer course of illness, are more prone to violence, homelessness, and poor adherence to treatments—the time to use the level of "awareness of illness" as a subtype and/or dimension in the *DSM* is long overdue. This is especially true when we look at the research on motivational enhancement therapy (MET) or Motivational Interviewing, and cognitive behavioral therapy (CBT), which, along with long-acting injectable medications, are clearly the treatments of choice for such individuals.

When a psychiatrist or other mental health professional meets someone with schizophrenia and does the initial evaluation, the question of whether the individual is like half of all persons with schizophrenia and related disorders—who do not understand they are ill and, as a consequence, refuse treatment and services—should *always* be asked.

||||||||||||||||||||||||||||||||||||||||||||||||||||||||||||||||||||||||||||||||||||||||||||||||||||||||||||||||||||||||||||||||||||||||||||||||||||||||||||||||||||||||||||||||||

The first step after making a diagnosis is to...identify whether the person...has anosognosia. Once we do that, we can then choose a different path toward stabilization and recovery—one that employs science-proven communication skills and medications designed to help persons with poor insight and poor adherence to treatment.

||||||||||||||||||||||||||||||||||||||||||||||||||||||||||||||||||||||||||||||||||||||||||||||||||||||||||||||||||||||||||||||||||||||||||||||||||||||||||||||||||||||||||||||||||

Such patients fight with well-meaning clinicians and family members who are trying to engage them in the interventions that can give them a chance at recovery. They (understandably, because they are certain nothing is wrong with them) toss out prescriptions, appointment cards, and advice regarding their disorder and treatments.

We know how to engage such persons in treatment—the science exists. The first step after making a diagnosis is to do a careful assessment of insight into illness and identify whether the person being evaluated has anosognosia. Once we do that, we can then choose a different path toward stabilization and recovery— one that employs science-proven communication skills and medications designed to help persons with poor insight and poor adherence to treatment.

20

Henry

On April 23, 2007, while standing on a sidewalk and helping a woman put her groceries on a bus, my brother Henry was hit by a car and died at the scene. There's a videotape of what he did, taken by the bus company, though I don't yet have the strength to watch it.

That was so like him. Although often lost in delusional thoughts and distracted by hallucinations, he was aware of people around him, especially those in need, and he cared.

That was not what he or I had planned for. When I first wrote about this, only two months after his death, I was much too close to my loss and mourning to know what good could possibly come from it all—but I had to trust that someday something would.

Saying Goodbye Twice

Standing at the lectern, looking out at the people who had come to Henry's funeral, I was struck once again by what a full life he had had. His friends filled the church, prompting several of my family members—who had had very little contact with Henry after he became ill 25 years before—to say things like "I had no idea he had this many friends!" and "I never knew his life was so full."

As they met and spoke to more and more of his friends over the course of that day and the next, some in my family expressed deep remorse and sadness that they had missed out on so much of his life. I didn't feel that sadness because I had not — my brother and I were very close and loved each other's company immensely. Henry was my hero.

The reason I had this relationship with Henry while others in our family did not is *not* because I am a better person; I am no saint. The reason is that after he first became ill, I was somehow able to mourn who he had been before, while most of my brothers and sisters (there are nine of us) seemed unable to.

At first, I know we all felt it — it was impossible to accept that he was no longer there in the way he had been. Handsome, kind, and loving with a magical sense of humor, he would never become the person we all had envisioned he would — a loving husband and father, a responsible caregiver and successful man.

When he became ill with schizophrenia, we all longed for the "old Henry" and made little room in our hearts for the "new Henry." He had the same problem.

For the first five years of his illness he, like us, was stuck on the plan he had had for the future, and he became depressed that what he had planned now seemed impossible to attain. Prior to becoming ill, he had always worked, gone to university and had girlfriends. That was over now. Not until he had mourned his old vision for the future did he discover that the core of the old Henry was still there and realize that new plans needed to be made.

The last year of his life he was especially happy. This is not some wishful revisionist delusion on my part — it is confirmed by all that were close to him. He had many friends; he worked odd jobs with his friend "Pops," and his girlfriend Mary had become a big part of his life.

Mourning When Mental Illness Strikes

The research is clear on the importance of mourning. By mourning what has been lost, you open your eyes to all that is still there. Moreover, you open your eyes and heart to new possibilities.

In a review of the research on literature we published in the spring of 2007 in the *Annals of General Psychiatry,* my colleagues and I found that people with schizophrenia who had successfully mourned were less likely to feel suicidal. Studies of family members of people with schizophrenia have found that those relatives that who have mourned the loss of the way things used to be are less likely to be critical of their mentally ill loved ones, and feel less burdened and stressed.

Some research findings are intuitive—they just make sense. This is one of those instances. I saw that same transformation in my brother and experienced the improvement in his hopefulness about his future and our relationship. I've seen it repeated time and again in the patients and families I have worked with this last 25 years.

Closing One Door Opens Another

It is like any other major change in life. When you mourn, you feel sad because you are saying goodbye to what was and what you hoped would be. But by doing this, you feel at peace—and even happy—as you say hello to what is and what *can* be. I have counseled many families and also consumers on the importance of going through this process. Families that successfully mourn are able to let go of their anger at their loved ones. They learn to separate the illness from the person. Communication gets healthier, and even the course of illness can improve because of the lessened tensions between family members.

But I never before experienced the stark truth of this wisdom so completely as I did when my brother died. Now that he is gone, I find I have no regrets.

I cherish countless good memories of him. I remember our nearly constant laughter together, his helping me build an outdoor fireplace in my home which crackled with flame and heat for my family earlier this evening, his giving me permission to write about him, the pride he felt in me and I in him, and so much more.

I recall our many conversations, how often he would ramble, and how it would be hard for me to listen. Despite all, he would always end by saying, "You're my baby brother, and I love you."

After Henry became ill, many things changed. But not the fact that he was smart, handsome, kind, and loving. Or how he could make me laugh — splitting-your-gut laughter — in any situation, even at our mother's funeral! He usually did it with kindness and reverence for the feelings of other people — except for those rare instances later in life when the illness got the best of him. Because he felt less inhibited, he was far funnier than he was prior to becoming ill and he knew it.

Many people have written to me to offer their condolences, to share their good memories of Henry, and to wisely say how lucky I was to have him as my older brother. They are right.

But they left out one vital thing, a lesson I learned anew as I reflected on the seemingly insurmountable task of saying goodbye to him all over again. I was especially fortunate that I was able to mourn after he first became ill — to say goodbye to what I had hoped for — so that during these past 25 years, I could laugh with him, make new good memories with him, and realize just how lucky I was to be his "baby brother."

Henry worked with me to get well and our relationship was a good one. He helped many people through his example, his influence on my thinking, and his willingness to let his story be told in my books and articles. We will never know how many lives he saved and how many people with poor insight he helped to recover.

I have received many letters from kind souls telling me he had that impact—I am sure there are many more who have not written.

I have much to be grateful for.

Acknowledgments

I am grateful, first and foremost, to my children Tatiana, Robinson and Aniceto. Thank you for your love, patience and sacrifice while I revised this book. Thank you most for making me laugh even when I was "grumpy man" and for making me feel like the luckiest man on earth. I love you more than you can know. I am and always will be your Dad and Papa.

My thanks also to Bob and Jason for your support and help while writing this book and with our other work together. Thanks to LEAP faculty for pitching in and giving LEAP seminars when I could not.

Since the publication of the first edition of this book, I have given lectures to tens of thousands of family members, mental health professionals, consumers, attorneys and judges in the U.S., Canada, and overseas. The response to the message and lessons in this book has been truly overwhelming. With each invitation to speak and every e-mail and phone call I receive, I am reminded again that I am bound to my readers by much more than a book. The shared experiences, words of appreciation, and lessons I have learned from these contacts have been invaluable and inspired me to write this 20th anniversary edition.

Once again, I especially want to thank the many people with mental illness who have opened up to me over the past 30 years and taught me about their experience. Thanks also to the students I have supervised. Without their enthusiasm for understanding the people whose care they were entrusted with, I would never

234 • I AM NOT SICK – I DON'T NEED HELP!

have had to translate research findings into practical advice they
could use in their clinical work.

Many organizations have supported the research described
in this book. I want to thank them for their support and for their
commitment to research on serious mental illness. My thanks to
the National Alliance for Research on Schizophrenia and Affective
Disorders (NARSAD), the Stanley Research Foundation, the
Scottish Rite Foundation, the National Institute of Mental Health
(NIMH), and the National Alliance on Mental Illness (NAMI).

And once again, *muchos gracias a mi hermano*. Thank you for
letting me tell our story and for being the kindest and most supportive older brother a person could ask for. Your perseverance
and sense of humor set a standard I continue to strive to meet. I
miss you, despite feeling your presence every day.

Literature Cited

Amador XF, Flaum M, Andreasen NC, Strauss DH, Yale SA, Clark SC, & Gorman JM. Awareness of illness in schizophrenia and schizoaffective and mood disorders. *Archives of General Psychiatry*, 51: 826-836. 1994.

Amador XF & David AS (Eds.) *Insight and Psychosis: Awareness of Illness in Schizophrenia and Related Disorders.* Oxford University Press, 2005.

Amador XF & Gorman JM. "Psychopathologic domains and insight in schizophrenia." *Psychiatric Clinics of North America,* 20: 27-42, 1998.

Amador XF, "Closing the Gap between Science and Practice," *Civil Rights Law Journal,* in press.

AmadorXF, Strauss DH, Yale SA, Flaum M, Endicott J, & Gorman JM. Assessment of Insight in Psychosis. *American Journal of Psychiatry,* 150: 873-879. 1993.

Amador XF, Barr W.B.; Economou, A.; Mallin, E.; Marcinko, L.; Yale, S."Awareness defects in neurological disorders and schizophrenia."*Schizophrenia Research,* 24(1-2): 96-97, 1997.

Amador XF, Harkavy Friedman J, Kasapis C, Yale SA, Flaum M, & Gorman JM. "Suicidal behavior and its relationship to awareness of illness." *American Journal of Psychiatry,* 153:1185-1188, 1996.

Amador XF & Seckinger RA. "The assessment of insight." *Psychiatric Annals,* 27(12): 798-805, 1997.

Amador XF & Strauss DH. Poor insight in schizophrenia. *Psychiatric Quarterly,* 64: 305-318. 1993.

Amador XF, Strauss DH, Yale SA & Gorman JM. Awareness of Illness in Schizophrenia. *Schizophrenia Bulletin,* 17:113-132, 1991.

Bartko G, Herczog I & Zador G. Clinical symptomatology and drug compliance in schizophrenic patients. *Acta Psychiatrica Scandinavica,* 77: 74-76. 1988.

235

McEvoy JP, Applebaum PS, Geller JL, Freter S. Why must some schizophrenic patients be involuntarily committed? The role of insight. *Comprehensive Psychiatry*, 30: 13-17. 1989.

Caracci G, Mukherjee S, Roth S & Decina P. Subjective Awareness of Abnormal Involuntary Movements in Chronic Schizophrenic Patients. *American Journal of Psychiatry*, 147: 295-298. 1990.

Cuesta MJ & Peralta V. Lack of Insight in Schizophrenia. *Schizophrenia Bulletin*, 20:359-366. 1994.

Flashman LA, McAllister TW, Saykin AJ, Johnson SC, Rick JH, Green RL. Neuroanatomical Correlates of Unawareness of Illness in Schizophrenia. From the Neuropsychology & Brain Imaging Laboratories, Dept. of Psychiatry, Dartmouth Medical School, Lebanon, NH & New Hampshire Hospital, Concord, NH 03301. Presented at the *Biennial Meeting of the International Congress on Schizophrenia Research*, Santa Fe, New Mexico, April 20, 1999

Ghaemi NS & Pope HG, Jr. Lack of Insight in Psychotic and Affective Disorders: A Review of Empirical Studies. *Harvard Review of Psychiatry*, May/June: 22-33. 1994.

Greenfield D, Strauss JS, Bowers MB & Mandelkern M. Insight and Interpretation of Illness in Recovery from Psychosis. *Schizophrenia Bulletin*, 15: 245-252. 1989.

Heinrichs DW, Cohen BP & Carpenter WT, Jr. Early Insight and the Management of Schizophrenic Decompensation. *Journal of Nervous and Mental Disease*, 173: 133-138. 1985.

Kampman O, Lehtinen K. Compliance in psychoses. *Acta Psychiatrica Scandinavica*. 100(3): 167-75, 1999.

Lysaker PH, Bell MD, Milstein R, Bryson G & Beam-Goulet J. Insight and Psychosocial Treatment Compliance in Schizophrenia. *Psychiatry*, Vol. 57, 1994.

Lysaker PH, Bell MD, Bryson G & Kaplan E. Neurocognitive function and insight in schizophrenia: support for an association with impairments in executive function but not with impairments in global function. *Acta Psychiatrica Scandinavica.* 97(4): 297-301, 1998.

McEvoy JP, Appelbaum PS, Geller JL & Freter S. Why Must Some Schizophrenic Patients be Involuntarily Committed? The Role of Insight.*Comprehensive Psychiatry* 30: 13-17, 1989.

McEvoy JP, Apperson LJ, Applebaum PS, Ortlip P, Brecosky J & Hammill K. Insight in schizophrenia: Its relationship to acute psychopatho-logy.*Journal of Nervous and Mental Disorders*, 177: 43-47, 1989.

McGlashan TH, Levy ST & Carpenter WT, Jr. Integration and Sealing Over: Clinically Distinct Recovery Styles from Schizophrenia. *Archives of General Psychiatry*, 32: 1269-1272, 1975.

McGlashan TH & Carpenter WT, Jr. Does attitude toward psychosis relate to outcome? *American Journal of Psychiatry*, 138: 797-801, 1981.

Michalakeas A, Skoutas C, Charalambous A, Peristeris A, Marinos V, Keramari E & Theologou A. Insight in Schizophrenia and Mood Disorders and its Relation to Psychopathology. *Acta Psychiatrica Scandinavica*, 90: 46-49, 1994.

Mohamed S, Fleming S, Penn DL & Spaulding W. Insight in schizophrenia: its relationship to measures of executive functions. *Journal of Nervous & Mental Disease.* 187(9): 525-31, 1999.

Morgan KD, Vearnals S, Hutchinson G, Orr KGD, Greenwood K, Sharpley R, Mallet R, Morris R, David A, Leff J & Murray RM. Insight, ethnicity, and neuropsychology in first-onset psychosis. *Schizophrenia Research*, 36(1-3): 144-145, 1999.

Smith TE, Hull JW & Santos L. The relationship between symptoms and insight in schizophrenia: a longitudinal perspective. *Schizophrenia Research.* 33(1-2): 63-7, 1998.

Swanson C, Jr., Freudenreich O, McEvoy JP, Nelson L, Kamaraju L & Wilson WH. Insight in Schizophrenia and Mania.*The Journal of Nervous and Mental Disease*, 183: 752-755, 1995.

Takai A, Uematsu M, Ueki H, Sone K & Kaiya Hisanobu. Insight and its Related Factors in Chronic Schizophrenic Patients: A preliminary Study. *European Journal of Psychiatry*, 6: 159-170, 1992.

Voruganti LN, Heslegrave RJ & Awad AG. Neurocognitive correlates of positive and negative syndromes inschizophrenia. *Canadian Journal of Psychiatry*. 42(10): 1066-71, 1997.

Wciorka J. A Clinical Typology of Schizophrenic Patients: Attitudes towards their Illness. *Psychopathology*, 21: 259-266, 1988.

Wilson WH, Ban T & Guy W. Flexible System Criteria in Chronic Schizophrenia. *Comprehensive Psychiatry*, 27: 259-265. 1986.

World Health Organization, Report of the International Pilot Study of Schizophrenia. Geneva: World Health Organization Press. 1973.

Young et al. Medication adherence failure in schizophrenia: a forensic review of rates, reasons, treatments, and prospects. *Journal of the American Academy of Psychiatry and the Law*, 27(3): 426-44, 1999.

Young DA, Davila R, Scher H. Unawareness of illness and neuropsychological performance in chronic schizophrenia. *Schizophrenia Research*, 10: 117-124. 1993.

Young DA, Zakzanis KK, Baily C, Davila R, Griese J, Sartory G & Thom A. Further Parameters of Insight and Neuropsychological Deficit in Schizophrenia and Other Chronic Mental Disease. *Journal of Nervous and Mental Disease*, 186: 44-50. 1998.

Research on Cognitive Therapy for Schizophrenia

Kemp R, Hayward P, Applewhaite G, Everitt B, David A: Compliance therapy in psychotic patients: a randomized controlled trial. *BMJ* 1996; 312: 345–349.

Kemp R, Kirov G, Everitt B, Hayward P, David A: Randomized controlled trial of compliance therapy: 18 month follow-up. *Br J Psychiatry* 1998; 172: 413–419

Kline N, Li C, Lehmann H, Lajtha A, Laski E, Cooper T: Beta-endorphin-induced changes in schizophrenic and depressed patients. *Arch Gen Psychiatry* 1977; 34: 1111–1113

McGorry PD, Yung AR, Phillips LJ, Yuen HP, Francey S, Cosgrave EM, Germano D, Bravin J, McDonald T, Blair A, Adlard S, Jackson H. Randomized controlled trial of interventions designed to reduce the risk of progression to first-episode psychosis in a clinical sample with subthreshold symptoms. *Arch Gen Psychiatry* 2002; 59: 921–928

Mosher LR, Menn AZ: Community residential treatment for schizophrenia: a two-year follow-up. *Hosp Community Psychiatry* 1978; 29: 715–723

O'Donnell C, Donohoe G, Sharkey L, Owens N, Migone M, Harries R, Kinsella A, Larkin C, O'Callaghan E: Compliance therapy: a randomised controlled trial in schizophrenia. *BMJ* 2003; 327: 834

Sensky T, Turkington D, Kingdon D, Scott JL, Scot J, Siddle R, O'Carroll M, Barnes TRE: A randomized controlled trial of cognitive-behavioral therapy for persistent symptoms of schizophrenia resistant to medication. *Arch Gen Psychiatry* 2000; 57:165–172

Tarrier N, Yusupoff L, Kinney C, McCarthy C, Gledhill A, Haddock G, Morris J. Randomised controlled trial of intensive cognitive behaviour therapy for patients with chronic schizophrenia. *BMJ* 1998; 317: 303–307

Tarrier N, Wittkowski A, Kinney C, McCarthy C, Morris J, Humphreys L: Durability of the effects of cognitive-behavioural therapy in the treatment of schizophrenia: 12-month follow-up. *Br J Psychiatry* 1999; 174: 500–504

Tarrier N, Kinney C, McCarthy E, Humphreys L, Wittkowski A, Morris J: Two-year follow-up of cognitive-behavioral therapy and supportive counseling in the treatment of persistent symptoms in chronic schizophrenia. *J Consult Clin Psychol* 2000; 68: 917–922

Wagemaker H, Jr., Cade R: The use of hemodialysis in chronic schizophrenia. *Am J Psychiatry* 1977; 134: 684–685

Recommended Books

Surviving Schizophrenia (Fourth Edition) E. Fuller Torrey. HarperCollins, 2001

Crazy: A Father's Search through America's Mental Health Madness. Pete Earley, Putnam, 2006

Insight and Psychosis: Awareness of Illness in Schizophrenia and Related Disorders. Amador XF & David AS (Eds.) Oxford University Press, 2005

Cognitive-Behavioral Therapy of Schizophrenia. David G. Kingdon and Douglas Turkington. The Guilford Press, 1993.

When Someone You Love is Depressed: How to help without losing yourself. Laura Epstein and Xavier Amador. Fireside, 1998

The Day the Voices Stopped: A Memoir of Madness and Hope. Ken Steele and Claire Berman. Basic Books, 2001

Recommended Resources

Advocacy & Professional Organizations

LEAP Foundation for Research to Practice (LFRP)
www.LFRP.org

The LEAP Foundation for Research to Practice is a non-profit 501(c) (3) dedicated to serving family caregivers of persons with serious mental illness (SMI) and addiction, mental healthcare professionals, criminal justice professionals, and others involved in the care, recovery, and safety of persons suffering from these disorders.

Our primary mission is to educate about the unmet needs of persons with mental illness and addiction who have anosognosia---persons who do not understand they have an illness and could benefit from treatment and services.

Closing this gap between science and practice – what research has found to be effective versus what people commonly do to help persons with poor awareness of their disorders – is a core goal of the LEAP Foundation.

The LEAP Foundation provides science-based education and training and other support to organizations and individuals wishing to learn about these disorders, anosognosia and the LEAP program. Training and certifying LEAP trainers is among our top priorities. The LEAP program and approach focuses on creating trusting relationships that lead to engagement and acceptance of treatment and services.

National Alliance on Mental Illness (NAMI)
www.NAMI.org

In my experience, NAMI is probably still the best source for support and information about serious mental illness. It was founded in 1979 by families of mentally ill people who were frustrated by the lack of services, treatment, research, and education available for mentally ill people and their relatives. It has become an influential and important advocacy group with local chapters in almost every major city as well as many smaller towns. Many chapters offer free "Family-to-Family," "In Our Own Voices" and, "Peer-to-Peer" programs that I highly recommend. Some chapters have hotlines you can call during a crisis or just to get information about services in your area. NAMI also offers excellent books and pamphlets about mental illness.

AL-ANON Family Groups
www.al-anon.org

Al-Anon members are people, just like you, who are worried about someone with a drinking problem. Family members have the opportunity to learn from the experiences of others who have faced similar problems. In fact, members run the groups and there is no fee to attend meetings. Al-Anon may be listed in the white pages of your local telephone directory. Cities with local information services are listed on their website. Many of those listed post meeting information on their websites. For meeting information in Canada, the US, and Puerto Rico you can call 1-888-4AL-ANON (1-888-425-2666).

Alcoholics Anonymous (AA)
www.AA.org

Alcoholics Anonymous is an international fellowship of men and women who have had a drinking problem. It is nonprofessional, self-supporting, multiracial, apolitical, and available almost everywhere. There are no age or education requirements. Membership is open to anyone who wants to do something about his or her drinking problem. There is no fee to attend. The only requirement for membership in AA "is a desire to stop drinking."

The Treatment Advocacy Center (TAC)

The Treatment Advocacy Center is a national nonprofit organization dedicated to eliminating barriers to the timely and effective treatment of severe mental illness. The organization promotes laws, policies and practices for the delivery of psychiatric care and supports the development of innovative treatments for and research into the causes of severe and persistent psychiatric illnesses, such as schizophrenia and bipolar disorder.

The National Mental Health Association (NMHA)
www.NMHA.org

The National Mental Health Association is another effective nonprofit organization that addresses many aspects of mental health and mental illness. With more than 340 affiliates nationwide, NMHA works to improve the mental health of all Americans, especially the 54 million people with mental disorders, through advocacy, education, research, and service.

Depression Awareness, Recognition, and Treatment (D/ART)
National Institute of Mental Health
5600 Fishers Lane
Room 10-85
Rockville, MD
Phone: (800) 421-4211

This organization can give you good general information about depression, its signs and symptoms, and the latest in treatment options. D/ART publishes some excellent booklets and brochures about depression that you can request.

American Association of Suicidology
2459 South Ash
Denver, CO 80222
Phone: (303) 692-0985

This organization offers a variety of printed suicide prevention materials, primarily for use in schools and other institutional settings. However, they can also refer you to suicide hotlines and support groups in your area.

American Psychological Association
750 1st Street, N.E., Washington, D.C. 20002
Phone: (202) 336-5500

American Psychiatric Association
1400 K Street, N.W., Washington, D.C. 20005
Phone: (202) 682-6066

These last two organizations are the national associations of the professions of psychology and psychiatry, respectively. If you contact them, they can send you information about serious mental illnesses and their treatment, as well as refer you their qualified members in your area. The American Psychological Association also publishes fact sheets (*Facts About Schizophrenia*, etc.) that are very informative.

Informative Websites

Treatment Advocacy Center
www.psychlaws.org.

The National Institute on Mental Health
www.NIMH.org

www.Schizophrenia.com.
www.reintegration.com
www.schizophreniadigest.com
www.bipolarmagazine.com
www.bipolar.com

Praise for the First Edition

I Am Not Sick, I Don't Need Help!
Helping the Seriously Mentally Ill Accept Treatment

At last we have a volume for those individuals most closely associated with the mentally ill. In a very readable fashion, Dr. Amador addresses the nature of patients' unawareness of their illness and their need for treatment. He also clearly outlines the relevant research and gives clear prescriptions to help families and therapists deal with patients' obliviousness to their condition. I strongly recommend this to families and therapists of individuals with serious mental illness.

— **AARON T. BECK, M.D.,** *Emeritus Professor of Psychiatry, University of Pennsylvania, Department of Psychiatry*

This is the first book to address the elephantine question running roughshod over families of individuals with schizophrenia and bipolar disorder: *Why won't the sick person take his/her medicine?* Amador, a psychologist who has a brother with schizophrenia, has pioneered research on poor insight into illness, a.k.a. anosognosia, for the past decade and is an acknowledged authority on it. He blends clinical vignettes skillfully with his erudition, and the resulting mix is both edible and edifying. Most important, Amador provides families and mental health professionals with a concrete, step-by-step plan to improve awareness of illness. This book fills a tremendous void in the literature on schizophrenia and bipolar disorder.

— **E. FULLER TORREY, M.D.,** *Author, Surviving Schizophrenia*

Looking back, the strangest part was not the omnipresent government agents, the agonizing radiation weapons, or even my own super hero-like capabilities. What frightens me most is that my manic depression gave me an immovable certainty that it was the world around me that was convulsing but that my perception and judgment of it were unaltered. Thinking of this time leaves me frustrated and embarrassed as well as apprehensive that it might come again. I read Dr. Amador's book and felt better. First, he concretely and understandably establishes that most denials of treatment are but manifestations of the illness and that it is the illness that is the enemy. Dr. Amador then presents a powerful game plan for penetrating, or at least circumventing, sickness induced lack of insight that will maximize the cooperation with treatment of those affected. When I first became ill, I wish this book had been in the hands of someone who cared about me.

—**JONATHAN STANLEY, JD,** *Asst Dir, Treatment Advocacy Center and a consumer diagnosed with Bipolar Disorder*

There are several publications that address best practices for clinicians treating persons with schizophrenia. These are written from the perspective of the practitioner. There are a few books written from the perspective of the consumer or of the family member, but these do not incorporate the values of clinical insights, particularly those reflecting recent research findings. The great value of *I Am Not Sick, I Don't Need Help!* is that it incorporates both the consumer's perspective and that of the clinician. It finds common ground, pointing out where the consumer and his/her clinician can work together in partnership. It is practical, easy to read, and hopeful. I highly recommend it to anyone interested in helping those who, like myself, live with the condition we call schizophrenia.

—**FREDERIC J. FRESE III, Ph.D.,** *Summit County Recovery Project and a consumer diagnosed with Schizophrenia*

Of the myriad of problems presented by serious mental illness, Dr. Amador has focused on the single most critical factor. Breakthroughs in treatment will not be effective unless we deal with medication noncompliance and the related issue of poor insight into illness. Dr. Amador takes this issue on in *I Am Not Sick, I Don't Need Help!* and deals with it head-on, providing vital information and practical advice for both families and therapists of patients with schizophrenia and bipolar disorder. This book will be immensely helpful to anyone dealing with the problems of medication noncompliance and poor insight.

—**MICHAEL FLAUM, M.D.,** *Director of Mental Health, State of Iowa*

This is a wonderful book bringing together the personal experiences of a psychologist and a lay person who has a relative with serious mental illness. Dr. Amador's research and clinical experience makes this book a rich source of information and practical advice. It is one of the salutary characteristics of our culture that people who experience pain convert that pain into something productive. People who are victimized by, stressed by, and dismayed by serious mental illness will find this book enormously helpful. It contains information about new research and concrete advice that will be of enormous help to both the families of the seriously mentally ill and to the mental health professionals who care for them.

—**HERBERT PARDES, M.D.**, *President, New York-Presbyterian, The University Hospital of Columbia and Cornell, and former Director of the National Institute of Mental Health*

I Am Not Sick, I Don't Need Help! is essential reading material for family members battling with their mentally ill loved ones about the need for treatment. Dr. Amador provides an insightful, compassionate, and practical guide for handling the frustration and guilt that inevitably arises when dealing with a sick individual who, by virtue of their illness, is completely unaware of the need for treatment. What makes this book especially poignant is Dr. Amador's inclusion of his own personal account of his lifelong struggle with his own brother who suffers from schizophrenia, as well as his detailed presentations of patient cases. He does an exceptional job summarizing the compelling science behind poor insight, or anosognosia, clarifying that the loved one's lack of insight is not a product of a psychological defense mechanism, but is a result of the very brain dysfunction that underlies the illness. Practical tips on how to help a loved one with poor insight accept treatment or how to proceed with civil commitment, if necessary, make this book especially useful.

—**MICHAEL B. FIRST, M.D.**, *Editor, Diagnostic and Statistical Manual of Mental Disorders, Fourth Edition (DSM-IV)*

This is a well-written and must-read practical guide for those facing serious mental illness in a loved one, friend, or colleague. Delusions and psychotic thinking are quite beyond our everyday experiences, so it is not surprising that most people are at a loss about how to approach and obtain help for someone with serious mental illness. Those with psychosis may not even recognize that their own behavior and function is disturbed, let alone that they need treatment. If only the ailment were a stomachache rather than a malady in the part of the brain that distinguishes normal from abnormal!

—**DOLORES MALASPINA, M.D.,** *Professor of Psychiatry, Columbia University College of Physicians and Surgeons and Director, Clinical Neurobiology in Medical Genetics*

Lack of insight in people with schizophrenia and bipolar disorder is the major cause of many of the worst aspects of their illness, and may be the most recalcitrant since it is difficult to treat someone who thinks that nothing is wrong. Dr. Amador has spent the better part of two decades conducting research on this topic and has been the world's most influential scientist in this important area of work. In this book, he prescribes detailed interventions to help families and therapists deal with lack of insight and the many difficulties it causes people with major mental illness. Yet Amador is not an academic preaching from an ivory tower. His poignant personal experiences with people with schizophrenia, including his brother and close friend, are laced throughout this thoughtful, moving, and indispensable book. *I Am Not Sick, I Don't Need Help!* is an essential guide to anyone who knows, loves or treats someone with schizophrenia or bipolar disorder.

—**RICHARD KEEFE, PH.D.,** *Professor of Psychology in Psychiatry, Duke University Medical Center and author of Understanding Schizophrenia*

It is uncommon to find books that bring together the latest findings in psychiatry research with relevant and practical clinical advice. Even less common are those that do so in a readable and engaging fashion, for both families and mental health professionals. Dr. Amador accomplishes all of the above in *I Am Not Sick I Don't Need Help!*

—**ROBERTO GIL, M.D.,** *Director, Schizophrenia Research Unit at Columbia University and the New York State Psychiatric Institute.*

There is probably no more difficult or more important responsibility for a family member in our society than meeting the needs of a mentally ill child, sibling or close relative. Daily life can be a struggle and the future impenetrable with uncertainty. Dr. Amador has taken up the challenge of guiding the family member in order to bring a better life to the afflicted patient and the responsible relatives. The unique combination of sensitivities he brings to this task reflect both his life experience as a sibling of an afflicted brother and his many years of broad clinical practice.

Reflecting his own profound empathy and insight, the book is a guide to the shocked, bewildered and too often hopeless close relative.

It is no mere compendium of generalizations. It is a practical, step-by-step, program for achieving understanding and even expressing love in a situation where that love is difficult to convey.

His is a remarkable achievement and a great public service. Many lives of patients and their loved ones could be enhanced, often immeasurably if copies of this book were given to the families of every patient who begins to show signs of psychosis. As people use this book, it will mark the beginning of a sound remediation and even rehabilitation.

— **CONNIE LIEBER,** *President, National Alliance for Research on Schizophrenia and Depression*

I Am Not Sick, I Don't Need Help! addresses one of the toughest and most emotional problems in delivering mental health services.

Dr. Xavier Amador and Anna-Lisa Johanson tackle this challenge by drawing on their own painful personal experience. The book offers a sensitive presentation of a practical, clinically sound, approach to getting a severely ill person to accept needed treatment.

Written in a respectful tone, the book provides clear, concrete guidance to families and professionals. Skillful use of case examples enlivens the text, which is filled with difficult "real world" situations. The focus throughout is on building mutual understanding and trust, so involuntary treatment can be avoided, if possible.

I hope this book will be widely read. It gives us a much-needed and long overdue common ground for helping people in crisis.

— **LAURIE FLYNN,** *Former Executive Director, National Alliance for the Mentally Ill (NAMI)*

I hope you will be as impressed as I am with this book's approach to treatment for persons with serious mental illness. I strongly applaud Dr. Amador for working out these treatment strategies and for the sage advice he gives for persons involved in what continues to be one of the most challenging and perplexing arenas in modern health care.

In this book, Dr. Amador lays out a specific plan of attack that addresses this difficult problem. It is an effective strategy for finding common ground that can be used to build trust and cooperation for mutually addressing the problems of the patient. The justification and description of the "listen-empathize-agree-partnership" approach rings true to this person who "has been there." Particularly valuable is the recommendation that clinicians and relatives not openly challenge the beliefs of the mentally ill person. Unfortunately such challenging is still quite common and is frequently justified by the thought that "you should not buy into the belief system" of a delusional person.

Such thinking among mental health providers is misguided. What is important, particularly during the initial stages of interaction is that the professional afford dignity to those in his care. How important it is to communicate respect.

In addition to describing effective strategies for dealing with mentally ill persons and providing a list of helpful resources, Dr. Amador provides delightful anecdotes that emphasize his main points and illustrate his suggestions. These serve as excellent mechanisms for tying his recommendations to the realities of trying to help mentally ill persons.

— FREDERIC J. FRESE III, Ph.D., *Clinical Assistant Professor of Psychology in Psychiatry, Northeast Ohio University's College of Medicine and a consumer diagnosed with Schizophrenia*

CREATING STRONG RELATIONSHIPS

Quick Start Guide

Listen   Reflect back without judgment, reactions, or contradictions

Empathize   Express empathy for feelings coming from delusions, anosognosia & desires

Agree   Find areas of agreement—abandon your goal of agreeing the person is sick

Partner   Move forward to achieve common goals you **can** partner on

❧

Delay   Delay giving hurtful and contrary opinions—redirect conversation

Opinion   With humility, give your opinion in a way that respects the person's perspective

Apologize   For acts & interactions that feel disrepectful, hurtful or disappointing

You may have noticed that the last three tools also spell out an acronym: D.O.A. I listed them this way to make this tool easier to remember and because I believe our relationships are indeed Dead On Arrival when we don't use the tools above.

About the Author

Dr. Amador is an internationally sought-after speaker, clinical psychologist, professor at State University of New York, the Director of the LEAP Institute and Foundation and author of eight books.

In 2010, Dr. Amador and his LEAP program were featured in the PBS's NOVA series, *This Emotional Life*. Dr. Amador's expertise has made him a regular contributor to the Today Show and a featured guest of ABC's *Good Morning America, Prime Time Live, CBS This Morning, NBC Nightly News, 60 Minutes, CNN, Dateline, ABC's World News Tonight, Fox News, The New York Times, The Wall Street Journal, USA Today* and many others.

Dr. Amador has been a consultant to numerous companies and government agencies including the National Institute of Health. His forensic cases include: the Unabomber, PFC Lynndie England, the Elizabeth Smart kidnapping, and the trials of Zacarias Moussaoui and accused 9/11 co-conspirator Ramsi bin al Shibh.

Dr. Amador has over 35 years' experience working with adults, families, and couples. He lives in New York.

Previously, Dr. Amador was a professor in the Department of Psychiatry at Columbia University, College of Physicians & Surgeons; on the Board of Directors of the National Alliance for the Mentally Ill (NAMI); Director of Research at NAMI; and the Director of Psychology at the New York State Psychiatric Institute.

Dr. Amador has published over 100 peer-reviewed scientific papers, and many other publications that have been translated into more than 20 languages.

Dr. Amador was co-chair of the last text revision of the Schizophrenia and related disorders section of the *DSM IV-TR* (often referred to as the "Psychiatrists' Bible").

CREATING STRONG RELATIONSHIPS

LEAP® (Listen-Empathize-Agree-Partner®) shows clinicians, family members, and law enforcement professionals how to quickly gain the trust of someone who is angry or paranoid. It gives you the tools you need to persuade someone in "denial" about mental illness to accept treatment and/or voluntarily comply with your requests. It grew out of Dr. Xavier Amador's:

- Successful struggle to convince his brother Henry, who was diagnosed with schizophrenia, to take the medications prescribed for him.

- Thirty-five years of hands-on clinical experience with patients who lacked insight.

- Experience gained from hundreds of LEAP seminars involving tens of thousands of clinicians, family members, and law enforcement.

- Twenty-five years of clinical research supported by the NIMH, Stanley Research Foundation, American Psychiatric Association, and NARSAD.

Since the book *I Am Not Sick, I Don't Need Help!* was published, hundreds of thousands have learned LEAP from the author and LEAP Institute faculty worldwide.

For more information, please visit

www.LEAPInstitute.org